Praise for *The Healing Power of* NATUREFOODS™

"Americans are increasingly aware that food quality determines our health. For 35 years, Susan has understood this and knows that food is usually the best medicine for what ails us. In *The Healing Power of* NATUREFOODS, she brings this wealth of knowledge together in one impressive book and tells you how to select, prepare, store, and use medicinally more than 50 familiar foods. Her tasty and inventive recipes promise boundless pleasures for your everyday table. This is a must-read for vegetarians, nonvegetarians, and anyone interested in vibrant health and nourishing food from an outstanding culinary instructor who writes from the heart."

Neal Barnard, MD, Founder and President
Physicians Committee for Responsible Medicine
Author of *Breaking the Food Seduction*

"NATUREFOODS is a book you'll treasure for years to come. Dr. Jones has superbly bridged the gap between the highly technical world of nutritional science and the real world of everyday eating and health practice. This book is readable, reliable, and entertaining, abounding with simple yet delicious recipes. Susan participated in a national television talk show in our restaurant, extolling the virtues of our menu, recipes, and the advantages of raw foods in general. She is a shining example of the benefits of a living-food lifestyle. Kudos to Susan."

Tolentin Chan
Quintessence Restaurant, New York City

"Reading *The Healing Power of* NATUREFOODS is an important step on the road to optimal health. You will learn how to choose the best foods to create a healthy and happy life. Read it and add years to your life and life to your years!"

Joel Fuhrman, MD
Author of *Eat to Live*

"NATUREFOODS is a gem. It's filled with sound food advice, practical culinary tips, and the essential keys to create a life filled with vibrant health and the celebration of natural foods. If you need some inspiration to upgrade your diet, this is the book for you!"

Shera Raisen, MD
Raisen Integrative Medicine, Santa Monica, California

"In a very understandable and entertaining way, Dr. Jones crystallizes all the reasons we've been told to 'eat our fruits and vegetables.' She has diligently reviewed the medical and scientific literature on these important foods so that it's clear how much control we have over our health by simply choosing the proper foods, some of which will come as a pleasant surprise. Well done, Dr. Jones!"

Brian S. Boxer Wachler, MD, Director
Boxer Wachler Vision Institute, Beverly Hills, California

"Do you wish you could achieve your natural weight, have abundant energy and a clear mind, look years younger, disease-proof your body, and find inner peace? Now you can! NATUREFOODS holds the simple keys to help rejuvenate your body, mind, and spirit. Susan presents a powerful, healthy approach for anyone who's rushed, stressed, sick, or simply desires radiant health and vitality. This book is an excellent guide, providing both sound nutritional direction and easy-to-prepare recipes. We thoroughly enjoyed NATUREFOODS and recommend it highly."

Denise Cook, PhD, and Chuck Cook, MD
Portland, Oregon

"Susan reminds us that all nutrients needed by the body are available in unadulterated whole foods. It couldn't be any simpler; the basis of life is eating a variety of natural, colorful foods as close to the way nature made them as possible. *The Healing Power of NATUREFOODS* now holds a prominent place in our library at the NHA."

Lynn Grudnik, Executive Director
National Health Association
Editor, *Health Science*

"Susan Smith Jones brings together the latest and most dramatic findings about all the foods we eat and drink. In a wonderfully lucid presentation, she makes a banquet of facts into an attractive, manageable meal of nourishing information. I will enthusiastically recommend NATUREFOODS to my patients."

Edgar Maeyens, MD
Coos Bay, Oregon

"Susan Smith Jones knows that eating food closest to its natural state creates a remarkable energy exchange between food and body. The result is a transformation to optimal vitality. Read *The Healing Power of NATUREFOODS* and find out which 50 colorful foods increase energy levels, boost immune function, dispel depression, support emotional stability, enhance vision, beautify skin, improve digestion, and sustain overall great health."

Gabriel Cousens, MD
Author of *Rainbow Green Live-Food Cuisine*

"If you are exhausted, struggling with health issues, and futilely battling your weight; if you suffer from insomnia, asthma, and allergies; if you find you just do not have the vitality and optimism you once had; or if you simply desire to calm a stressed nervous system, restore immunity, prevent illness, and live a happier and healthier life, then *The Healing Power of NATUREFOODS* is the perfect book for you. In easy-to-understand language, Susan presents the healthiest foods and recipes to transform your body, your health, and your life. Enthralling and cogently readable!"

Leslie Van Romer, DC
Author of *Food Power, You Power*
Sequim, Washington

"*The Healing Power of* NATUREFOODS is a thorough and practical guide for anyone seeking wellness through the wonderful medicinal power of food. Susan's extensive recommendations are well researched, concise and, most important, easy to implement. Her delicious recipes fit perfectly into my busy schedule. Overall, this book is essential for everyone who cares about being disease-free and radiantly healthy."

Nancy S. Schort, DDS
Santa Monica, California

"In *The Healing Power of* NATUREFOODS, Susan Smith Jones provides the reader with a better understanding of the specific advantages of the plant kingdom as an excellent source of nourishment. Her material is based on the perfect balance of scientific knowledge, nutritional wisdom, and long-standing culinary experience."

Elson M. Haas, MD, Founder and Director
Preventive Medical Center of Marin
Author of *The New Detox Diet*

"In *The Healing Power of* NATUREFOODS, Dr. Susan Jones blends the joy of eating with solid advice about health. It's primary reading for those who believe, as I do, that good health starts in the kitchen. If you apply its contents in your life, it is guaranteed to bring you tremendous rewards of vibrant health and a renewed zest for life."

Ben Kim, DC
Life Essentials Health Clinic, Barrie, Ontario

"Read *The Healing Power of* NATUREFOODS and say goodbye to low energy, poor digestion, aches and pains, extra pounds, and disease. Instead, say hello to mental clarity, a lean, trim body, renewed vigor, and better overall health. This book offers a gift of knowledge, inspiration, practical wholefood recommendations, and easy-to-prepare, scrumptious recipes."

Rev. John Strickland
Unity

"Dr. Susan Jones is a frequent guest on my radio show and a wonderful example of living by God's natural health laws. Fortunately, we all now have access to her wealth of knowledge and experience in *The Healing Power of* NATUREFOODS. Whether you're age nine or ninety-nine, you'll welcome her guidance on how to heal your body, mind, and spirit. This is my favorite health book."

Louie B. Free
Host of the radio talk show *Brainfood from the Heartland*

"Build up your defenses with *The Healing Power of* NATUREFOODS—a medically sound, reader-friendly, and helpful book that elucidates diet's role in wellness and disease prevention. Outstanding!"

Maj. Gen. Peter J. Gravett, USA (Ret.)

"Susan's popular health articles have been appearing regularly in national magazines for over 35 years. Her most recent discoveries are presented in a sensational new book—*The Healing Power of NatureFoods*. In this easy-to-read book, Susan combines the latest medical research with her wisdom as a caring, nutritionally aware health expert to create a clear, optimistic guide to staying younger far longer. With topics ranging from antioxidant-rich foods that protect arteries and cells to strategies to boost immunity, beautify skin, improve vision, and enhance endurance, mental clarity, and overall wellbeing, she pieces together the multiform clues to longevity and vitality. Let Susan show you how to age gloriously with dignity and radiant health."

Olin Idol, ND, CNC
Vice President of Health, Hallelujah Acres

"For years, Susan Smith Jones's articles have been among the most popular in our magazine. She's a dedicated health educator with a talent for translating vital, current nutritional information into elegant, understandable prose. Luckily, Susan has now put much of her vast knowledge into *The Healing Power of NatureFoods*, a cutting-edge, scientific, and practical guide for using the power of colorful foods to heal your body, conquer disease, and stay healthy. This remarkable book should be savored by anyone interested in living a long and vibrant life in body, mind, and spirit. It's full of amazing facts and sound advice that our entire staff is reading with great interest!"

Cindy Saul
Editor/publisher, *phenomeNEWS*

"Can we actually live on a diet of primarily fresh fruits and vegetables? Absolutely! I have been thriving on such a diet for over 20 years. In fact, this diet is solely responsible for my overcoming a medically incurable disease and helping me reclaim my life. Read *The Healing Power of NatureFoods* and learn about these delicious, healing foods."

David Klein
Publisher of *Living Nutrition*

"In *NatureFoods*, Susan presents a stunning synthesis of the importance of eating whole, natural foods. I've been fortunate to have Susan as my personal culinary instructor several times each year for the past 25 years, and I've also attended many of her motivating and inspiring workshops. Thankfully, I now have her invaluable health and food knowledge in this enjoyable book; it's the best health gift I could give myself and all of my friends and loved ones. Terrific!"

Jamie S. Carr
Rancho Santa Fe, California

"I thoroughly enjoyed *NatureFoods*! It has given me an appreciation for how the simple foods I now choose to eat can make a profound difference in how I feel. Susan's easy-to-prepare, delicious recipes are perfect for my busy lifestyle. I highly recommend this book to anyone who wants to look and feel his or her best."

Angela Colasanti
Pottstown, Pennsylvania

"*The Healing Power of* NATUREFOODS is the most empowering book I've ever read on how to prevent disease and create youthful vitality. Susan has a gift of taking complex research and scientific studies and making the material easy to understand and incorporate into one's life. Everyone needs to read this gem of a book over and over again. I keep extra copies on hand to give as gifts."

Lisa Ray, skin specialist and salon owner, Skin Premiere
West Los Angeles, California

"Susan has been my private culinary instructor for 15 years and, thankfully, I now have NATUREFOODS as my constant companion when Susan is not here. One of the greatest food blessings I learned from Susan is the importance of simple meals. Because of her ingenuity, I now make countless quick, healthful meals for my family. This superb book will change your life for the better. It is immensely inspiring!"

Donica Beath
Eugene, Oregon

"*The Healing Power of* NATUREFOODS is illustrious. It's your passport to health and vitality for years to come. Everyone who eats should dig right in. This book contains vital dietary information you simply should not miss!"

Charles M. Taylor, Minister, CEO/President
Stars Unlimited Coaching, Miami, Florida

"In addition to being an insightful guide to the best salutary foods with simple suggestions on how to prepare healthy meals, *The Healing Power of* NATUREFOODS also offers a bonanza of research-based nutritional pearls. Since reading this book and implementing Susan's practical advice and delicious recipes, we are healthier and more energetic than ever in our lives."

Susan and Bill Kulick
North Bend, Oregon

"Whether you want to enhance weight loss, to look younger, or to heal a serious illness, *The Healing Power of* NATUREFOODS is the best place to come for a long visit. Susan presents timeless, life-saving information and an easy path to optimum health through eating natural foods. This is an important and eminently readable book for our new century of self-care. Thanks, Susan, for leading the way."

Dave and Alice Neighbors
West Los Angeles, California

"*The Healing Power of* NATUREFOODS is user-friendly, informative, and timely. Kudos to Dr. Jones, who has produced an indispensable resource that is uniquely vital and beneficial. I highly recommend this book to everyone who desires to expand their health options, enliven their inner healer, and live forever young. Simply and elegantly, Susan sheds new light on age-old health wisdom and offers an abundance of sound nutritional advice along with easy-to-prepare recipes."

Nick Lawrence
Radio/TV talk-show host

THE
HEALING
POWER
OF
NATURE
FOODS

Also by Susan Smith Jones, PhD

CELEBRATE LIFE!

BE HEALTHY~STAY BALANCED

WIRED TO MEDITATE

CHOOSE TO LIVE FULLY

LEARN TO LIVE A BALANCED LIFE

MAKE YOUR LIFE A GREAT ADVENTURE

A FRESH START: REJUVENATE YOUR BODY

VEGETABLE SOUP/THE FRUIT BOWL
(co-authored with Dianne Warren)

To order, contact:
www.SusanSmithJones.com

Hay House Titles of Related Interest

Eating in the Light: Making the Switch to Vegetarianism on Your Spiritual Path,
by Doreen Virtue, PhD, and Becky Prelitz, MFT, RD.

The True You Diet: The revolutionary diet programme that identifies your unique body chemistry and reveals the foods that are right for YOU,
by Dr John Briffa

Your Secret Laws of Power: The Modern Art of Healthy Living,
by Alla Svirinskaya

* * *

The products above are available at your
local book store, or may be ordered by visiting:

Hay House UK: **www.hayhouse.co.uk**
Hay House USA: **www.hayhouse.com**®
Hay House Australia: **www.hayhouse.com.au**
Hay House South Africa: **orders@psdprom.co.za**
Hay House India: **www.hayhouse.co.in**

THE HEALING POWER OF NATURE FOODS

50 Revitalizing SuperFoods & Lifestyle Choices to Promote Vibrant Health

Susan Smith Jones PhD

HAY HOUSE

Australia • Canada • Hong Kong • India
South Africa • United Kingdom • United States

Published and distributed in the United Kingdom by:
Hay House UK Ltd, 292B Kensal Rd, London W10 5BE. Tel.: (44) 20 8962 1230;
Fax: (44) 20 8962 1239. www.hayhouse.co.uk

Published and distributed in the United States of America by:
Hay House, Inc., PO Box 5100, Carlsbad, CA 92018-5100. Tel.: (1) 760 431 7695 or (800) 654 5126;
Fax: (1) 760 431 6948 or (800) 650 5115. www.hayhouse.com

Published and distributed in Australia by:
Hay House Australia Ltd, 18/36 Ralph St, Alexandria NSW 2015. Tel.: (61) 2 9669 4299;
Fax: (61) 2 9669 4144. www.hayhouse.com.au

Published and distributed in the Republic of South Africa by:
Hay House SA (Pty), Ltd, PO Box 990, Witkoppen 2068. Tel./Fax: (27) 11 467 8904.
www.hayhouse.co.za

Published and distributed in India by:
Hay House Publishers India, Muskaan Complex, Plot No.3, B-2, Vasant Kunj,
New Delhi – 110 070. Tel.: (91) 11 4176 1620; Fax: (91) 11 4176 1630. www.hayhouse.co.in

Distributed in Canada by:
Raincoast, 9050 Shaughnessy St, Vancouver, BC V6P 6E5. Tel.: (1) 604 323 7100;
Fax: (1) 604 323 2600

A catalogue record for this book is available from the British Library.

ISBN 978-1-4019-1600-8

Printed and bound in Great Britain by TJ International, Padstow, Cornwall.

"I dwell in Possibility."
— Emily Dickinson

"Each patient carries his own doctor inside him."
— Albert Schweitzer

*"The natural force within each one of us
is the greatest healer of all diseases."*
— Hippocrates

*"The doctor of the future will give no medicine,
but will interest his patients in the care of the human frame,
in diet, and in the cause and prevention of disease."*
— Thomas A. Edison

*"If we want to know how to maintain wellness,
we must first understand how we are made,
how our body is designed to heal itself,
and what foods God created for our bodies to function properly."*
— Dr. George H. Malkmus

*"Nothing will benefit health
and increase the chances for survival of life on Earth
as much as the evolution to a vegetarian diet."*
— Albert Einstein

*"You see things; and you say, 'Why?'
But I dream things that never were; and I say, 'Why not?'"*
— George Bernard Shaw

* * *

This book is joyfully dedicated,
in loving memory, to my mother, June.
As proud as you always were of me,
I was even more proud of you.
Through your invincible courage,
resplendent spirit, and shining example,
you taught me how to love deeply,
live fully, and celebrate life.
I will love you always and forever.

It also is lovingly dedicated to God—
for the gift of life and the panoply
of colorful wholefoods,
and to everyone striving
to live healthful, balanced, halcyon lives.

And to you, dear reader,
I salute your great adventure.
May you be well nourished
by healthful foods and lots of love.

* * *

MENU

I. HORS D'OEUVRES

Foreword   3
Conversion chart   6
Introduction   7
Healthful Eating Tips   13
10 Simple Steps for Success   17

II. ENTRÉES

50 NatureFoods: Part I   21
  Almonds   22
  Apples   23
  Asparagus   24
  Avocados   25
  Bananas   26
  Beans   28
  Beets   29
  Bell Peppers   30
  Blueberries   31
  Broccoli   32
  Brussels Sprouts   33
  Cantaloupe   35
  Carrots   36
  Celery   37
  Chili Peppers   38
  Cinnamon   39
  Coconut   40
  Cranberries   41
  Cucumbers   42
  Figs   43
  Flaxseed   45
  Garlic   46
  Ginger   48
  Goji Berries   49
  Grapefruit   50
  Green Leafy Vegetables   51
  Kale   54

III. INTERMISSION
Healing Power of Raw Foods & Fresh Juices   59

IV. More ENTRÉES
50 NATUREFOODS: Part II   71
   Kiwi   71
   Lemons   72
   Medicinal, Culinary Herbs & Spices   74
   Mushrooms   75
   Oats   76
   Onions   78
   Oranges   79
   Parsley   80
   Parsnips   81
   Pears   82
   Persimmons   84
   Pomegranates   86
   Raspberries   87
   Sea Vegetables   88
   Sesame Seeds and Tahini   90
   Spinach   92
   Strawberries   94
   Sunflower Seeds   95
   Sweet Potatoes   96
   Tea   97
   Tomatoes   98
   Walnuts   99
   Watermelon   100

V. RADIANT HEALTH AT A GLANCE
How NATUREFOODS Keep You Healthy   104

VI. RECIPES
42 NATUREFOOD RECIPES   109

NUT & SEED MILKS
Sunflower Seed Milk   110
Sesame Milk   110
Almond Milk   111

JUICES & BLENDS
Orangey Apple Zinger Juice   111
Skin-Beautifying Cocktail   112
Warm Apple Cider   112
Carotenoid Cocktail   113
Heavenly Cantaloupe Cocktail   113
Beet Veggie Juice   113
Rejuvenating Parsley Pear Blend   114
Watermelon Ginger Refresher   114
Phytonutrient Power Drink   115

SMOOTHIES
Perfectly Persimmon Smoothie   115
Chocolate Sweet Potato Smoothie   116
Kiwi Melon Smoothie   116
Glorious Grapefruit Juice/Smoothie   117
Cranberry Grape Plunge   117
Coconut Fruit Smoothie   118
Strawberry Banana Smoothie   118
Pomegranate Fruit Smoothie   119

VEGETABLE SALADS
Crunchy Broccoli Bell Salad   119
Savory Cucumber Fennel Salad   120
Corny Onion Salad   120

FRUIT SALADS
Banana Bites   121
Citrus Cinnamon Delight   121

DRESSINGS & DIPS
Grapefruit Tahini Dressing   122
Fresh & Luscious Lemon Dressing   122
Orange Balsamic Vinaigrette   123
Groovy Guacamole   123
Sensational Salsa   124
Tahini Salsa Dressing   124

Spicy Sprouted Hummus 125
Mellow Mushroom Gravy 126
Cranberry Pineapple Relish 126

FRUIT & NUT TOPPINGS
Vanilla Orange Cream 127
Omega-3 Walnut-Flax Topping 127
Fabulous Fig Sauce 128
Pear Cashew Cream Topping 128

SOUPS & BISQUE
Sweet Pepper & Almond Soup 129
Chilled Berry Blueberry Soup 129
Spicy Sweet Potato Bisque 130
Golden Gazpacho Soup 130

VII. MOTIVATIONAL TOOLS
Setting Up Your Healthy Kitchen 133
Afterword 139

VIII. RESOURCES
Recommended Reading, References &
  Other Resources 145
Books & Audio Programs
  by Susan Smith Jones 149
Ongoing Education & Support 151
9 Tips to Create More Joy & Less Stress 153
Commitment to Health 155

Gratitude 156
About the Author 157

I

HORS D'OEUVRES

FOREWORD

by Lendon H. Smith, MD
author of *Happiness Is a Healthy Life*

I have known Dr. Susan Smith Jones for over three decades. She is a fellow Smith, but that's not the reason I always appreciate seeing her radiant face on the covers and pages of health magazines. She says all the things I want to say; and she says them sooner, more clearly, and more cogently.

Susan faces the same dilemma all health writers face. Presenting up-to-date health information acquired through diligent research and personal experience is not enough to bring about a diet and health revolution. Unless you can motivate readers to *use* that information, to make the changes necessary to transform their diets and living habits, success will be limited. Fortunately, Susan is a master motivator, and you will soon see how delightfully satisfying it is to eat better, to become more active, and to start kicking some of your bad habits. No one else offers such fruitful information in a reader-friendly and engaging style.

Many of us have long suspected a deeper purpose—call it divine genius—for the brilliantly colorful beauty of fruits and vegetables. Now there is research to prove that these foods attract us for good reason—they are overflowing with the precise nutrients we need to achieve radiant health and youthful vitality.

NATUREFOODS is a timeless, much-needed food and healthful living guide that can help you realize your highest health potential at any age and help you

3

avoid the negative consequences of the poisons in our environment, not-always-perfect genes, and other unfortunate facts of modern life. Sadly, most people think it's "normal" to experience a host of ongoing ills—weakened vision, stiff joints, an unreliable bladder, an inability to sleep, and more—as we age. How much better it would be to live disease-free for about a century and then to go quietly in your sleep.

MY WIFE WAS ONCE IMMOBILE for a couple of months with a sciatica-like problem, so I bought and fixed the meals. My menus were enough to motivate her to get well. I tried to push us both into more raw foods and less meat. Actually, I found it was easy to shop; I just stayed around the periphery of the supermarket and did not enter the aisles where the denatured packaged and processed foods lay in wait for uninformed consumers.

I think I know why most people of my generation (I'm in my later years) have lived long and reasonably healthy lives. We were not exposed to the many pollutants, herbicides, and toxic chemicals so common today. We also did not have the "advantage" of modern food marketing techniques that process and deplete natural foods so that they can sit on the grocers' shelves forever. Since World War II, the rates of most diseases have increased: heart disease, cancer, diabetes, obesity, asthma and allergies, ADD/ADHD, arthritis, and autoimmune diseases such as lupus. In addition, people are developing these degenerative diseases earlier in life.

Thankfully, scientific research has discovered natural, easy-to-understand solutions to most of these problems. The trouble is, they require that people change their eating and living habits. How can we get our population—especially those who already are suffering from ill health—to make much-needed, healthful changes? Adolescents think they are immune and immortal, middle-aged people feel their insurance will get them through, and the elderly figure, "What's the use, I'm too old to start now." Wrong! No matter what your age, you can start today by following the easy-to-understand guidance in this book.

I suggest that you read about a few foods at a time, study, ponder, and follow Susan's recommendations, and incorporate them into your lifestyle. Don't try to do too much at once, or try to totally overhaul your diet overnight. One step at a time is always the best approach.

When people ask me what to do about their ills—their constipation, their congestion, their headaches, their aches and pains, their disturbed sleep—my first question is: "What is your favorite food?" If people love a food so much they would kill for it, it represents an allergic-addictive situation. There is something in that food that has created an addiction. Susan can tell you how to get all of the nutrients you need from healthful food sources that don't cause dangerous addictions.

ONE OF THE BEST THINGS about Susan is her cheerful and enthusiastic personality. She knows how to turn you on to her style and methods even though you may be reluctant to take that first step. Once you are into her ways and you feel better, you will thank your lucky stars that you have this esteemed book as your guide.

Susan has included material on how foods devoid of nutritional value, if eaten on a regular basis, can cause a depressed, negative attitude—putting you in a foul, cranky, and onerous mood. I find that surly, grumpy people can become so self-centered that they no longer can even smile or nod a hello to their fellow human beings. My feeling is that people in that condition likely have not eaten well or exercised for days or weeks. My advice to them is to read this book and follow Susan's recommendations. As they start eating healthier foods—taking better care of themselves physically—their attitudes will change from negative to positive.

How simple is Susan's message? You can almost figure it out for yourself. Try to picture yourself as one of your ancestors ages ago, running through field and forest, eating as you go, cooking little, laughing a lot, and sleeping with one eye open. Some wild thing might eat you, but with your healthful diet and outdoor life, at least you'd know your body is healthy and, well, delicious—good enough to eat.

Happy foraging—in the store and in this book.

CONVERSION CHART

gram = 0.035 oz
kilogram = approx. 2.2 lb
litre = 35.2 fl oz

ounce/oz = 28 g
pound/lb = 454 g
gallon = approx. 3.8 l
foot = approx. 30 cm

cup = approx. 230 g
tablespoon/tbsp = approx. 15 g or 15 ml
teaspoon/tsp = approx. 5 g or 5 ml

Introduction

"Let food be your medicine and medicine be your food."
— Hippocrates

For 35 years, I've been a researcher, writer, teacher, lecturer, counselor, and lifestyle coach with an emphasis on holistic health, optimal nutrition, and living a balanced life. Known to many as the "Food Doctor", I've always looked to nature for the answers on how to be my healthiest. I don't use prescription drugs, and I believe that God has provided us with everything we need to be vibrantly healthy right into old age. In Genesis 1:29, we find the following passage:

> Then God said, "Behold, I have given you every plant yielding seed that is on the surface of all the earth, and every tree which has fruit yielding seed; it shall be food for you."

Following this sound advice will do wonders to help you create a vibrantly healthy and youthful body and rejuvenate your life. Eating whole- and live-food cuisine will enable you to tap into the miraculous healing power of creation.

Nature encourages health and balance. In nature's splendor we find the spirit of beauty within each of us and all of the food we need to radiate with a healthy glow—like the morning light or the sky at dusk. While the foods we eat are only one aspect of being healthy, diet is definitely an indispensable starting point. Statistics reveal that eight of the ten leading causes of death in North America are directly related to diet. That's a sobering statistic, especially when you consider that we are free to choose any foods we can afford. Nobody shoves the food down our throats. Many of us make the wrong food choices every day. By consuming foods we were never intended to eat, we set ourselves up to develop most of the common major diseases.

A few diehards who have successfully avoided learning anything about the nutritional research of the past 40 years may argue that a diet emphasizing whole, fresh, plant-based foods is radical or outlandish, but I challenge them to show *any* research that supports the consumption of the greasy, fat- and cholesterol-laden foods that so many Americans are consuming these days. Even Houdini could not escape from the fact that dairy and animal products, salt, sugar, refined carbohydrates, artificial colors and flavors, preservatives, and various "food" additives all are associated with problems. A diet of adulterated foods has been scientifically proven to increase the risk of heart disease, cancer, obesity, arthritis, and diabetes, to name a few.

"We have become so brainwashed," writes Dr. George H. Malkmus in his inspiring book, *God's Way to Ultimate Health: A Common Sense Guide for Eliminating Sickness Through Nutrition*, "that we think it is 'normal' to eat a meal of processed, adulterated foods from a tin can, cardboard box, or frozen dinner containing man-made chemical ingredients that can't even be pronounced by most people . . . but that someone who insists on eating food exactly as it was created by our Creator is a radical!" He goes on to say that it's imperative that we all consider the consequences of eating a diet consisting of artificial, nutritionally void foods that are grown, flavored, and preserved with synthetic, man-made chemicals. The price we pay for choosing these disease-causing foods is a life fraught with medical procedures such as endless rounds of prescription drugs, surgery, radiation, and chemotherapy. The astronomically expensive, highly inefficient medical establishment is in large part the inevitable result of our national dietary madness. In fact, opines Dr. Malkmus, those who profit from the processed food industry and medical procedures would like us to think that our current, woefully inadequate way of eating is *necessary* to sustain our bodies and maintain health.

Fortunately, there is another way of eating and living, one that heals our bodies, promotes radiant health, and rejuvenates our lives. Imagine, if you can, a life without ever feeling sick—without aches, pains, or fatigue. Imagine never getting colds or the flu or depression. Imagine waking up each day—bouncing out of bed—eager to experience life's great adventures with joy and élan. Imagine not being tempted by unhealthful foods or recreational drugs, or succumbing to noisome addictions. Imagine being your ideal weight and having people consistently praise you on how beautiful/handsome and youthful you look, and wanting to know about your diet and lifestyle. Imagine never needing to contend with cosmetic surgery. Imagine not needing to spend a penny on prescription drugs. If you can, imagine, also, feeling so vibrantly healthy that you only visit your doctor once a year or so to get an annual checkup. And imagine your doctor's surprise and delight when you show up feeling and looking younger than your previous visit. It is music to the ear to hear the doctor say that you are in superior health and have the physiology of someone 20 years your junior, and the doctor wants to learn from *you* what you're doing to be so healthy.

Nature is beckoning all of us to come back home—to "live by Nature's Laws", as my grandmother used to say. We need to choose foods that sustain life and feed the more than 70 trillion cells in the body with optimum nutrition.

IN THIS BOOK, YOU WILL DISCOVER the importance of eating "live-food" cuisine (made with raw food), which accelerates weight loss, facilitates healing, and restores youthful vitality. You also will learn how to make the best food choices to reduce your risks of heart disease, hypertension, diabetes, obesity, Alzheimer's, arthritis, common forms of cancer, premature aging, vision problems, and mental dysfunction. I'll also describe ways to increase your energy, joie de vivre, and sense of empowerment over your body and your life. You'll learn the importance of selecting a variety of colorful, antioxidant-rich, plant-based foods, preferably organically grown, as they do have more nutritional value. With each passing year, scientific studies are revealing more about the active components of plant-based foods called phytonutrients. Phytonutrients are chemical compounds in plants that act on human cells and genes to bolster your body's innate defenses against illness. Put simply, phytonutrients can save your life.

Antioxidants (non-vitamin nutrients that abound in some plant foods) are equally extolled for fostering radiant health. As a result of what is likely the largest antioxidant study in history to date, the U.S. Department of Agriculture (USDA) has produced a list of the 20 most antioxidant-rich foods. You already may have heard that blueberries rank high. But, if you are like me, some of the findings might surprise you. The study examined more than 100 types of fruits, vegetables, berries, nuts, and spices. Top food sources of antioxidants included artichokes, russet potatoes, and ground cloves. In the end, small red beans took the top spot, narrowly beating out wild blueberries as the food with the highest concentration of disease-fighting compounds per serving.

A prevailing but still controversial theory holds that antioxidants may benefit the body by providing protection against oxidation, a process that may be linked to conditions such as cancer, heart disease, and aging. Found most often in colorful produce, antioxidants are also available in powdered "green" supplements and pills.

The USDA study was published in the June 2004 issue of the *Journal of Agricultural and Food Chemistry*. Here's the full list, starting with the richest source of antioxidants: small red beans (dried), wild blueberries, red kidney beans, pinto beans, blueberries (cultivated), cranberries, artichokes (cooked), blackberries, prunes, raspberries, strawberries, Red Delicious apples, Granny Smith apples, pecans, sweet cherries, black plums, russet potatoes (cooked), black beans (dried), plums, and Gala apples.

So when in doubt about what foods to eat, elect to select colorful plant foods rich in phytochemicals and antioxidants, and eat them as close to the way nature made them as possible. You might consider copying this list of antioxidant-rich foods and keeping it in your wallet so you can pull it out when grocery shopping or conversing with friends and family.

For decades, my family, friends, and clients have come to me with specific physical conditions, ailments, and diseases, wanting suggestions on the best natural remedies. For example, recently I recommended blueberries to a friend because they can increase brain longevity through their ability to help release dopamine in the brain. For another client, one who has heart disease and cancer, I recommended spinach and kiwi because of their high levels of disease-fighting antioxidants and phytonutrients. A participant in one of my workshops was concerned about fibroid tumors, and I recommended pears because of their high content of certain minerals and fibers thought to help prevent fibroid tumors.

Throughout this book, you'll learn how to make good food choices instead of taking medicine and also how to select the best foods, kitchen appliances, and other health-promoting products that help disease-proof the body and make being radiantly healthy easy and fun. For easy reference, I'll list the foods in alphabetical order. Every food is backed by extensive research and my personal experience and instruction—teaching nutrition and healthful food preparation classes (cooked and live-food cuisine) for more than 25 years.

I HAVE HAD THE BLESSED OPPORTUNITY to witness recoveries of radiant health—body, mind, and spirit—by family, friends, and clients who simply made improved food choices, gravitating toward the foods recommended in this book. The key is to eat these salutary foods as close to the way nature made them as possible. In other words, adopting a colorful, fresh, whole-foods diet will profoundly change your life and, quite possibly, extend it!

By eating the foods suggested in this book, you will be able to heal your body, promote radiant health, and rejuvenate your life. I encourage you to make a commitment for 30 days—just one month—and incorporate as many of these foods as possible into your diet. In just one month, you will look better than you have in years and also will feel more youthful and empowered. What do you have to lose except some extra weight, aches and pains, ailments and diseases, and a negative attitude toward your body and life? I know you can do it. I believe in you and salute your great adventure. I hope to meet you in person somewhere along the way.

* * *

HEALTHFUL EATING TIPS

*"I look younger. My skin is more supple now
and I have fewer wrinkles than I did before eating raw."*

— Carol Alt

Supermodel, actress, author of *Eating in the Raw*

Before we begin with the first NATUREFOOD, let's briefly touch on the importance and benefits of a plant-based diet, since this book is all about emphasizing these salubrious high-fiber, plant-based foods.

Fiber fills you up. It's what makes foods filling without being fattening. The word itself simply means "plant roughage," like the skin of an apple, cucumber, or pepper, or the chewy part of oats. Fiber gives foods crunch, makes them substantial, and gives them staying power. Fiber promotes good digestive health, helps lower cholesterol and insulin levels, and reduces the risk of many cancers, including cancers of the breast and colon. Research shows that people who consume the most high-fiber foods are the healthiest, as determined by better waist measurements, lower insulin levels, and other markers of disease risk. Indeed, this is one of the key themes of this book—for anyone to consider his or her diet healthful, it must be predominantly composed of high-fiber, plant-based, natural foods.

In his groundbreaking book, *Breaking the Food Seduction: The Hidden Reasons Behind Food Cravings—and 7 Steps to End Them Naturally*, Neal Barnard, MD, president and founder of the Physicians Committee for Responsible Medicine, provides this poignant example of why fiber is so important for those concerned about their weight. Take a generous-sized tablespoonful (about 15 grams) of any sort of fat or oil. That spoon of grease, he says, has about 135 calories. The same quantity (weight) of carbohydrate or protein packs about 60 calories. But that same amount of fiber has essentially *no calories at all.* It fills you up at least as well as do fatty or high-protein foods, but you'll never see it on the scale. He reminds us that there is no fiber in eggs, bacon, sausage, yogurt, or any other animal-derived product. They aren't plants, and *only plant foods have fiber.*

Researchers have found that you can cut your calorie intake by a full 10% just by adding an extra 14 grams of fiber each day. (*J Pediatr Psychol* 2002 Sept; 27(6):531–40) Over the long run, that can really help trim excess pounds. In another study, researchers looked at the eating habits of a large group of people living in Alabama, California, Illinois, and Minnesota. The subjects all followed typical American diets, more or less, but some got more fiber than others. The difference wasn't huge: about 10 grams of fiber per day for those at the lower end, compared to about 20 for those who got the most fiber. But, even within that range, fiber made a noticeable difference on the scale. Those whose diets were richer in fiber weighed *eight pounds less,* on average, than those who got less fiber. (*Nutr Neurosci* 2002 Apr;#5(2):141–4)

To be as radiantly healthy as I talked about in the introduction, Dr. Barnard recommends that we shoot for 40 to 50 or more grams of fiber per day. My daily diet is teeming with at least 60 grams of fiber. Where do you find fiber? Simple. Four kinds of foods have plenty of healthy fiber: beans, vegetables, fruits, and whole grains, in that order. The more of these foods you build into your diet, the better off you are. A bowl of chicken soup with some noodles and a few vegetable bits doesn't have much fiber (about 1.5 grams). Chickens are not plants, so they don't have any plant roughage. Instead of chicken soup, choose a hearty bowl of split pea soup, which has 5 grams. Lentil soup has about 6 grams, and black bean soup has about 17 grams. Whether you prefer cooked foods or more live-food cuisine, you still can shoot for more fiber by adapting these plant-based foods to your daily food choices.

According to Barnard, if you want to control your appetite, achieve and maintain an optimal weight, and create a healthy body-for-life, you must aim for at least 40 grams of fiber each day. Eat that healthfully, and your body will thank you many times over.

For me, meal preparation is more of a joy when I have a little help from my friends—my kitchen gadget angels, who make my life easier! You can reduce your stress immeasurably by having a few culinary tools available that add to the beauty and diversity of the food and allow you to pull together healthful meals in minutes.

You don't need anything fancy or exotic, just good-quality everyday tools, such as various-sized sharp knives, whisks, a colander and sieve, mixing bowls and spoons, a salad spinner, a couple of Microplanes®, sprouting utensils, a food processor, a citrus reamer, a garlic press, cutting boards, high-quality cookware, a nut/seed grinder, a citrus juicer, a blender, and a top-quality fruit/vegetable juicer. As you will see in my recipes, these kitchen tools can make the difference between a good meal and a great one.

If there were only three kitchen appliances I could have, it would be the Total Blender, a Champion Juicer, and the Ionizer Plus filtered alkaline water machine. I use them several times each week to make a majority of dishes, including soups, smoothies, vegetarian "cheese" sauces, dressings, nut milks, "ice cream", purées, and nut butters.

* * *

10 Simple Steps for Success

"Whatever you can do or dream, begin it!
Boldness has genius, power, and magic in it."
— Johann Wolfgang von Goethe

Making a fresh start is so much easier when you have a solid plan for success. Here are 10 simple tips that will help you as you embark on a new, more healthful diet or improve your existing one. Let them inspire you as you choose a gloriously joyful path to the new you!

1. *Start strong.* Make the start date of your new program a special date. Clean your kitchen of unhealthful products, get your workout gear in order, and create a calendar where you can list your accomplishments. For example, on Day One, you might write that you walked for 30 minutes, meditated for 15 minutes, ate three pieces of fruit, and put a rejuvenation mask on before going to bed.

2. *Eat your morning meal.* Have breakfast within one hour of getting up in the morning. It stokes your metabolism and makes it easier to make healthier choices throughout the day.

3. *Curb your appetite.* Drink a large glass of water 15–20 minutes before a meal. Water detoxifies and rejuvenates your body and helps prevent overeating by making you feel full.

4. *Stop after 7:00 P.M.* To see rapid changes in your body shape, establish a habit of not eating after 7:00 P.M. To drop some weight quickly, stop eating

after 3:00 P.M., with the exception of a piece of fresh fruit, vegetable juice, or tea.

5. ***Feel your hunger.*** Snack only when hungry, not when bored, depressed, or tired. Remember, eat to live, don't live to eat. To prevent overeating, cultivate an appreciation for *quality* versus *quantity* in your food *and* lifestyle choices. Choosing quality over quantity enriches your life. Less is more to those who are wise and evolved. (One exception is my recommendation to eat *plenty* of leafy greens and most vegetables!)

6. ***Go light.*** When you're hungry and don't have much time, opt for low-calorie snacks that are quick and nourishing, such as fresh fruits and vegetables. If you crave more substance, add a few raw seeds or nuts, but no more than 1 oz. at a time if you have more than 10 pounds to lose.

7. ***Eat what you like.*** There are many delicious, healthy foods to choose, so don't eat what you don't like. Nothing makes a food program more difficult than forcing yourself to eat foods you don't care for.

8. ***Slow down.*** Eat slowly enough to give your body time to release the enzymes that tell your brain when you've had all you need. Inhaling food instead of eating consciously and deliberately causes indigestion and gas.

9. ***Don't give up.*** Falling off your health program once or twice does not mean the effort is hopeless. Simply acknowledge that you didn't eat wisely and get back on the program. If you make nutrient-rich whole foods (uncooked and unprocessed, whenever possible) the centerpiece of your diet, you will quickly learn to prefer these natural delights to less healthful choices.

10. ***Reward yourself.*** Treat yourself to a massage, a movie, or a new piece of clothing for each week that you faithfully complete your health program, lose weight, or accomplish some other goal.

* * *

II

ENTRÉES

50 NatureFoods
Part I

Little changes in your diet and lifestyle
will make big differences in the long run.

Now, let's take an in-depth look at 50 revitalizing NatureFoods that will put you on the path to better health, greater wellbeing, and youthful vitality. In addition to all of the unique nutritional benefits I will be describing, I occasionally mention a food's ORAC score. ORAC refers to the Oxygen Radical Absorbance Capacity, an analysis that is used to measure the total antioxidant power of individual foods. The higher a food's ORAC score, the greater its antioxidant capacity. Here are the ORAC units per 100 grams (about 3½ oz.) for a sampling of vegetables I will be describing: kale (1,770), spinach (1,260), brussels sprouts (980), broccoli florets (890), beets (840), red bell peppers (710), onions (450), corn (400), eggplant (390), and carrots (210). You'll want to strive to eat at least 3,000 ORAC units daily. I usually get between 5,000 and 6,000.

Please keep in mind that since my goal is to inspire you to transform your diet and zest for life, I am describing and emphasizing the very best benefits of the very best foods. However, I don't want to give the impression that you must precisely micro-manage every meal depending on how you are feeling that day, week, month, or year. Remember, while I am singing the praises of these best-of-the-best foods and describing their extraordinary health benefits, keep in mind that *all* fresh fruits, vegetables, legumes, raw nuts and seeds, and whole grains bring tremendous benefits. The unsurpassed nutrients and other qualities I describe for individual foods also can be found to varying degrees in *all* of the NATUREFOODS I recommend for a complete, overall healthful diet.

I have organized my list of foods and their recipes in alphabetical order so that after you've read everything, it will be easy to flip back through the book to find your favorites. Sound simple enough? Okay, let's get started.

Almonds

T his delicious nut makes a nutritious snack when you're hungry and on the go. Two ounces, or about 40 almonds, give you more than 50% of your daily requirement of magnesium, a mineral that's important for heart health. Almonds are also a good source of other heart-healthy nutrients, including calcium, vitamin E, potassium, folate (the plant form of folic acid), fiber, and monosaturated fat. In 2002, a study published in *Circulation* found that by eating about 2½ oz. of almonds per day for one month, participants significantly reduced their total cholesterol and lowered several other risk factors for heart disease as well. Another study suggested that eating almonds also may reduce the risk of colon cancer. An alkalizing nut, almonds are great as part of trail mix, ground and mixed in a salad, used as part of a raw pie crust, or made into raw almond butter. I eat six organic, raw almonds daily.

Try soaking almonds and other nuts and seeds overnight, drying them, and letting them germinate (sprout). During the germination process, each begins the transition from a nut or seed to a vegetable. This increases the life force and makes them easier to digest. Once soaked and dried, keep almonds refrigerated. They plump up and get larger after soaking; they are also easier to chew.

*See **Almond Milk** recipe on page 111.*

Apples

Eating "an apple a day" will most definitely help keep the cardiologist away. Current studies suggest that eating apples regularly reduces the risk of stroke and chances of dying from a heart attack. Apples lower total cholesterol and triglycerides. It's not clear which compounds are responsible, although flavonoids (which are antioxidants) and fiber are possibilities. Although whole apples have more fiber than juice, both forms probably benefit your heart. In a small clinical trial, researchers from the University of California at Davis found that drinking 12 oz. of apple juice daily was more effective than eating two apples per day at reducing oxidation of LDL ("bad") cholesterol, a heart-disease risk factor. Apples are the best fruit source of catechins, potent cancer-preventive substances. In fact, eating apples appears to decrease the risk of lung cancer, according to an epidemiological study from the Netherlands that was published in 2001. Still, the whole apple with the skin provides the highest level of nutritional value—a powerhouse of nutrients.

Apples also provide quercetin, which may inhibit prostate, lung, and liver cancer. And because of the high antioxidant activity, apples improve brain function and memory, too.

My favorite apple is the Fuji, but I also enjoy Gala, Golden Delicious, Granny Smith, Jonagold, Pink Lady, Braeburn, and Red Delicious. (Red Delicious are the highest in antioxidants.) I also incorporate raw, organic apple cider vinegar into my health program.

Apples can help ripen stone fruit, as well as other unripe fruits such as kiwis. Simply place the fruit in a loosely closed paper bag at room temperature with an apple. The apple will release ethylene gas, which accelerates ripening.

See **Warm Apple Cider** recipe on page 112.

Asparagus

A superior alkalizing vegetable, asparagus has the ability to quickly change the pH of the body, as evidenced by how rapidly you can smell it in your urine after you eat it. Asparagusic acid, a cyclic disulfate, is reported to be the main sulfur compound that gives asparagus its unique flavor and post-digestion urinary odor. You can "smell" it working when you urinate. According to Theodore A. Baroody, PhD, in his book *Alkalize or Die*, the odor is the result of the asparagus changing the body chemistry and eliminating wastes while it breaks down its constituents of nitrogen, sulfur, and ammonia. Prized as a springtime delicacy for centuries, this edible member of the lily family is now so widely cultivated that it is available in every season. Six spears have just 20 calories, but they contain 100 micrograms (mcg) of folate (25% of the adult recommended daily allowance, or RDA), 20 milligrams (mg) of vitamin C, and 200 mg of potassium.

Asparagus is also a powerful antioxidant. Antioxidants are substances that knock out free radicals, thus affording cellular protection. When healthy, the body eliminates most excess free radicals. Yet, with the poor foods people eat and the stresses most of us experience, these naturally protective antioxidants are overused and undersupplied by our bodies. Asparagus, particularly organically grown asparagus, contains the elements necessary to eliminate free radicals, the most important of which is the alkaloid asparagine. Also found in asparagus are vitamins A and C and other antioxidants that work synergistically in a perfect balance with the body. I eat asparagus spears raw just as I do celery or carrot sticks. I also enjoy them chopped into salads, juiced, and lightly steamed.

Avocados

Often referred to as "nature's butter", avocados are popularly known as the alligator pear because of the shape and rough skin of the most common variety. Other varieties of avocados are smooth-skinned, larger in size, and range in color from dark green to crimson. Avocados have more protein than any other fruit—approximately 2 grams per 4-oz. serving.

Rich in phytochemicals, this fruit (yes, avocado is a fruit) is the main ingredient in one of my favorite dishes—guacamole. You can spread it on whole-grain bread, mash it into baked sweet potatoes instead of butter or margarine, and even use it as a great hydrating facial mask. Avocados only have about a quarter of the total fat calories of dairy butter, compared by weight. And ounce for ounce, they provide more heart-healthy monosaturated fat, vitamin E, folate, potassium, and fiber than other fruits. In fact, a 4-oz. portion (about half of a medium-sized avocado) provides 500 mg of potassium and more than 16% of the RDA of folate; it also supplies 10% or more of the RDA for iron and vitamins C, E, and B6.

Avocados are rich in two phytochemicals: beta-sitosterol, an important phytochemical linked with lower cholesterol levels, and glutathione, an antioxidant that may offer protection against several cancers.

According to Susan Bowerman, RD, of the University of California at Los Angeles Center for Human Nutrition, avocados also exceed other fruits as a source of the potent antioxidant lutein. Lutein may safeguard your cardiovascular system from atherosclerosis (or hardening of the arteries) and prevent prostate cancer. It also protects your eyes from cataracts and from age-related macular degeneration.

If all of this doesn't get you excited about avocados, maybe this will: world-renowned nutrition expert David Heber, MD, PhD, says in his insightful book, *What Color Is Your Diet?*, that avocados were known as "testicle fruit" by ancient people in Central and South America and had a reputation as an aphrodisiac.

Avocados should be served raw; they have a bitter taste when cooked. A medium-sized California avocado contains about 30 grams of fat—almost twice as much as its Florida cousin—and more calories than any other fruit. If you desire to lose weight, limit your consumption to no more than one avocado per week because of their high-fat (albeit healthy fat) content. Avocados start to ripen only after being cut from the tree. Mature fruit can be left on the tree for six months without spoiling. Once picked, it will ripen in a few days.

See **Groovy Guacamole** recipe on page 123.

Bananas

Monkeys may be wiser than we think. Perhaps they know that their favorite food—the curvaceous banana—is one of the most nutritious tropical fruits. Both ripe and unripe bananas benefit the body. Fiber from green, unripe bananas dramatically reduces the "bad" (LDL) cholesterol and increases the production of "good" (HDL) cholesterol by up to 30%, as reported in the *Indian Journal of Experimental Biology*. (Effect of dietary fiber from banana on cholesterol metabolism. 22:550–554, 1984) The natural flavonoids in green, unripe bananas and plantains have been used to treat gastric and duodenal ulcers; bananas actually thicken the protective gastric mucosa. Do you have an upset stomach? Eat a ripe banana. This satisfying and stabilizing food soothes digestive disturbances such as constipation.

Bananas provide a wonderful source of readily available energy for young and old alike and may reduce fatigue. They also can help decrease the risk of stroke, relieve heartburn, prevent ulcers, and speed recovery from diarrhea. Bananas are a good source for baby's first food, especially because they are bland, easy to digest, and unlikely to produce allergies. But if eating a banana is not for you, mash it up and spread it on your face like a facial mask. The pulp from the banana makes a wonderful skin cleanser and hydrator.

As one of the leading fresh-fruit sources of potassium, bananas are in good supply all year long. One medium banana contains close to 400 mg of potassium, a mineral that plays a role in lowering blood pressure. A study on 17,000 adults indicated that higher potassium levels are associated with lower blood pressure. Bananas also contain the amino acid tryptophan, which stimulates the production of serotonin, a neurotransmitter that has a calming effect on the body.

With the possible exception of strawberries, no fresh fruit is higher in minerals than bananas. In addition to the high levels of potassium, a fresh banana also supplies 120 mg sulfur, 80 mg silicon, 33 mg of magnesium, and 26 mg of phosphorus, along with ample amounts of copper, chromium, iron, fluoride, manganese, selenium, and zinc. Sodium content is only 1 mg.

A medium (4-oz.) banana provides 45% of the RDA for vitamin B6. It also has 2 grams of dietary fiber, some of which is soluble fiber, instrumental in lowering blood cholesterol levels. Bananas contain about 100 calories each, mostly in the form of fruit sugar and starch. Keep a supply of ripe, peeled, and frozen bananas (in plastic freezer bags) available as they make the perfect ingredient to thicken and sweeten all kinds of smoothies. Frozen bananas on a stick also are delicious to eat as a cooling snack on warm or hot summer days.

Unless organically grown, most bananas are picked green and gassed with ethylene to speed their ripening. Allow them to ripen at home at room temperature, placing them in a closed paper bag to speed the process. When the skin is yellow and speckled with brown spots, the banana is ripe. The browner the skin, the higher the banana's sugar content.

*See **Banana Bites** recipe on page 121.*

Beans

Here is a food that unquestionably fits in the NATUREFOOD category. Legumes include fresh beans such as peas, green beans, and lima beans as well as lentils, chickpeas, black beans, and the entire dried bean family. Beans are not just a great source of fiber and protein; they also pack a powerful antioxidant punch. Vegetarians have long relied on beans as a healthier source of protein than meat. Surprisingly, until recently, few scientists had bothered to see if beans contained antioxidants—free-radical-destroying substances believed to help fight heart disease and cancer.

As mentioned in the Introduction, beans are particularly rich in antioxidants called flavonoids, the ones found in green, white, and black tea. Small red beans, red kidney beans, pinto beans, and black beans (in that order) are the richest in antioxidants, followed by yellow and white beans. The antioxidants are found in the bean coat, which is also where bean colors are found.

Most beans are about 1% fat, with soybeans being an exception. Soybeans are about 18-20% fat, of which 15% is saturated, 23% is monosaturated, and 58% is polyunsaturated. The primary isoflavones in soy are genistein and daidzein—which may help prevent cancer. However, one study found that anasazi, brown, black, navy, pinto, and turtle beans contain about as much or more genistein as soybeans. (*J Altern Compl Med.* 1997;3:7–12)

If you choose canned beans, always put the beans in a strainer and rinse them with cool water. This will eliminate about 40% of the added salt. Whether canned or fresh, beans are a great addition to toss in a salad or add to chili. Hummus, one of my favorite foods, is made from chickpeas, also called garbanzo beans. I also sprout beans so I can create raw-food hummus and other tasty treats. You even can grind dry beans into healthy flour using The Kitchen Mill™. *(See "Setting Up Your Healthy Kitchen" on page 133.)*

Okay, okay. It is true that beans can cause flatulence. This is because bacteria attack the indigestible matter that remains in the intestine. The following tips may work for you. Canned beans and mashed beans are less gas-producing. Eat beans frequently in small amounts so that your body can become accustomed to them. Soak beans before cooking; rinse, then boil them for 2 to 3 minutes; turn off the heat and let them soak for a few hours; rinse, add fresh water, and continue cooking. This boiling and soaking releases a large percentage of the indigestible carbohydrate in the beans, making them easier to digest. Pressure-cooking beans also reduces their gas-producing qualities; so does sprouting the beans.

See **Spicy Sprouted Hummus** *recipe on page 125.*

Beets

The sweet taste of the highly versatile beet belies its calorie content—a small one has only 22 calories. Beets are a good source of folate—an important B-vitamin that protects against heart disease and cancer. One cup of the beet tops, if eaten young and green, supplies 35 mg of vitamin C, 720 IU of vitamin A, 160 mg of calcium, 2.5 mg of iron, and a whopping 1,300 mg of potassium. My favorite way of utilizing the nutritious tops is by juicing them.

According to folklore, beets were believed to possess curative powers for headaches and other painful conditions. Even today, some health practitioners recommend beets to help prevent cancer and bolster immunity. I suggest using the juice of raw beets to speed convalescence and as a good overall body detoxifier and rejuvenator.

Antioxidants recently discovered in beets show promise for preventing heart disease, although research is preliminary. Betanin, one of these antioxidants, inhibited oxidation of LDL ("bad") cholesterol, according to a study published in 2001 in the *Journal of Agricultural and Food Chemistry.* This effect was shown in a test tube, but the researchers also found that people were able to absorb the antioxidants by consuming beet juice. Here's another reason to eat beets. According to a recent animal study, eating them significantly slowed the growth of skin and lung tumors.

There are so many ways to enjoy beets. They can be boiled and served as a side dish, pickled and eaten as a salad or condiment, or used as the main ingredient in borscht, a popular Eastern European cold summer soup. The most nutritious part of the vegetable—the greens—can be cooked and served like spinach or Swiss chard or, as mentioned above, juiced with other vegetables such as carrots, celery, cucumbers, and spinach. One word of warning, however, when consuming beets: They may make your urine and stools turn pink or even red after eating them. This is a harmless condition that occurs when betacyanin, the red pigment in beets, passes through the digestive system without being broken down. The urine and stools usually return to their normal colors after a day or two.

See **Beet Veggie Juice** recipe on page 113.

Bell Peppers

Sweet bell peppers, which are a dieter's best friend, range in color from green to yellow to orange to red, depending on their ripeness. Those picked while green will not become red, because peppers ripen only on the vine. Peppers grow sweeter as they ripen, which is the reason red ones are sweeter than yellow ones, which are sweeter than green ones. That's one of the reasons I prefer red bell peppers over the green ones. When green peppers ripen on the vine, they turn red and their vitamin content increases. So like some people and wines, peppers just get better with age.

A half-cup serving of peppers contains only 12 calories, but the vitamin content varies according to color. Ounce for ounce, peppers are a better source of vitamin C than citrus fruits. Because of this, I often eat them as a snack food, cut into strips (great dipped in guacamole or hummus), or eat one whole as I would savor an apple. Just one serving of green peppers provides more than 100% of the adult RDA for vitamin C, and red peppers provide 50% *more* of this antioxidant. They also are a great source of beta-carotene, fiber, folate, and vitamin B6, and are considered a top-ten antioxidant vegetable with an ORAC score of 710. (Actually, as any botanist will tell you, peppers are a fruit.)

A superb overall body alkalizer and healer, red bell peppers are an ideal ingredient that I juice or blend with other vegetables in my healthful beverage recipes. In addition, they are a breeze to roast and add to fresh hummus or other appetizing dips. One word of caution, however, before you fill your grocery basket with these delightful gems. They are also on the top-ten list of pesticide-laden vegetables when grown conventionally, so I highly suggest that you look for organic red, yellow, or orange bell peppers.

See **Sweet Pepper & Almond Soup** *recipe on page 129.*

Blueberries

Known as an excellent laxative, blood cleanser, and antioxidant, blueberries are the only food that have been shown to not just prevent, but actually *reverse,* abnormal physical and mental decline. Native to North America, blueberries have been part of the human diet for more than 13,000 years and rank among the best foods you can eat. I recommend eating them several times per week either fresh or, when out of season, frozen. I always have frozen organic blueberries on hand and use them when making smoothies. One cup of blueberries contains only 80 calories, and a whole pint gives you about 180 calories, so they're a dieter's good friend, too. Like all other foods, the calories in blueberries come from the *macro*nutrients—56 grams of carbohydrate, 1.5 grams of fat, and 2.7 grams of protein. But it is blueberries' *micro*nutrient content that packs the most impressive wallop.

Referred to as the "brain berry," blueberries are packed with anthocyanins (red pigments) that have been linked to prevention and reversal of age-related mental decline and anti-cancer effects. According to a study released in 2002 by Tufts University, anthocyanins in blueberries appear to be one of the most potent antidotes to oxidate stress, a process that ages you. The flavonoids in blueberries—catechin, epicatechin, myricetin, quercetin, and kaempferol—are extremely valuable for superior health. (Those flavonoid names are great words to bring up at your next prosaic dinner party or in your next *Scrabble* game.) Blueberries are to fruit what broccoli is to vegetables.

See **Chilled Berry Blueberry Soup** *recipe on page 129.*

Broccoli

Like the blueberry, broccoli is a supreme NATUREFOOD, and it is difficult to overestimate its healing powers. Broccoli has been proven effective as a food medicine against cancer, heart disease, and a host of other serious conditions. Two powerful cancer-fighting substances in this perfect food are sulforaphane and indole-3-carbinol. Sulforaphane gives cancer-causing chemicals a one-two punch. First, it destroys any carcinogenic compounds that you've ingested; then, it creates enzymes that eat up any carcinogens left over from that reaction. According to a recently released Johns Hopkins University study, sulforaphane kills the bacteria *H. pylori,* which causes ulcers and greatly increases the risk of gastric cancer. Indole-3-carbinol helps your body metabolize estrogen, potentially warding off breast cancer, a theory supported by epidemiological and clinical studies.

Besides being a superlative cancer-buster, broccoli also is a good source of beta-carotene, calcium, magnesium, vitamins B3 and B5, vitamin C, potassium, folate, chlorophyll, and fiber. The fiber in broccoli (4 grams in 1 cup) slows your body's release of blood sugar for long-lasting energy. Very low in calories and nutrient-dense, this cruciferous vegetable also may inhibit the reproduction of the herpes simplex virus. A substance called 13C, found in broccoli and related veggies, was found to be effective even though the herpes strain tested is resistant to current drugs.

Which food do you think has more protein—broccoli or steak? You would be wrong if you thought steak. Steak only has 5.4 grams of protein per 100 calories, and broccoli has 11.2 grams, almost twice as much. (*Eat to Live: The Revolutionary Formula for Fast and Sustained Weight Loss,* by Joel Fuhrman, MD) Unlike most of the calories in meat, which come from fat, most of the calories in green vegetables come from protein. (All calories come from fat, carbohydrate, or protein.) Here's some more food for thought. The biggest animals—elephants, hippopotamuses, giraffes, horses, gorillas, and rhinoceroses—all eat predominantly green vegetation. Where do they get the protein necessary to grow so big? They get it from the greens they eat. Obviously, greens, including broccoli, pack a powerful protein punch.

As you'll read more about later in the book, all protein on the planet is formed from the effect of sunlight on green plants. A cow doesn't eat another cow to get the protein necessary to build its muscles (which we call steak). The protein comes from the grass the cow eats. Most people mistakenly think they need to include animal products in their diets to ensure adequate protein intake. Fortunately, it's easy to get more than enough protein eating a plant-based, whole-foods vegetarian diet, which has the delightful side benefit of helping you avoid eating risky, cancer-promoting substances such as saturated fat. What's more, increasing the consumption of nutritious green foods such as broccoli is the key to achieving and maintaining safe, successful weight loss. There are so many ways to incorporate this quintessential food into your diet. I eat broccoli raw, occasionally lightly steamed, juiced, and in the form of sprouts, which magnifies broccoli's potent healing powers.

See **Crunchy Broccoli Bell Salad** *recipe on page 119.*

Brussels Sprouts

There are no prizes for guessing where brussels sprouts originated. The first were grown in large quantities in France and Belgium, particularly around the Belgian capital. As such, these crucifers are thought to be one of only two common vegetables that originated in northern Europe. (The other is kohlrabi.)

From 20 to 40 auxiliary buds grow close together along a tall, single stalk that's topped with small, cabbage-like leaves. Brussels sprouts aren't really sprouts at all; they are small cabbages.

Not surprisingly, brussels sprouts share many of the health benefits of cabbage. Like broccoli, cabbage, cauliflower, and other cruciferous vegetables, they contain chemicals that appear to protect against cancer. With an ORAC score of 980, they are rich in vitamin C (one cup of cooked brussels sprouts provides 100 mg) in addition to good amounts of folate, iron, potassium, and protein. Their health-promoting benefits don't stop here. Brussels sprouts also have high amounts of bioflavonoids and indoles, plant chemicals that protect against cancer in several ways. Bioflavonoids have an antioxidant effect that helps prevent cellular damage and mutation caused by the unstable molecules released when the body uses oxygen. Bioflavonoids, along with indoles and other plant chemicals, inhibit hormones that promote tumor growth. Indoles are particularly active against estrogen, the hormone that stimulates the growth of some breast cancers.

One study at the Fred Hutchinson Cancer Research Center found that men who ate three servings of cruciferous vegetables each week reduced their risk of prostate cancer by 41% compared with men who ate them only once per week. Cruciferous vegetables, it was noted, reduced prostate cancer risk even more than lycopene-rich tomatoes! These salutary green beauties also are rich in the pigments of chlorophyll, lutein, and beta-carotene and phytochemicals glucobrassicin (indole-3-carbinol), p-coumaric acid, D-glucaric acid, caffeic acid, ferulic acid, and alpha-lipoic acid—all wonderfully salubrious and beneficial for everyone interested in radiant health and vitality.

Low in calories and high in fiber, brussels sprouts become sweet and tender after a frost. Unfortunately, since our primary commercial supply of this vegetable comes from California's mild coastal area, brussels sprouts from the supermarket generally lack sweetness. If your region has frost, seek out local brussels sprouts. Prepare them for cooking by trimming them and cutting an "X" into the base of each one to enable the heat to penetrate their center more quickly and cook more evenly. Steam them just until tender, but still a vibrant green. I also half, quarter, or thinly slice them (makes a delicious hash), or for an elegant but time-consuming dish, separate each leaf. You also can add brussels sprouts to stir-fries and soups or to steamed, braised, or baked dishes. If you prefer live-food cuisine, as I do, include brussels sprouts as an ingredient in your medley of fresh vegetables for juicing.

Cantaloupe

One of my favorite fruits, cantaloupe is an excellent cleanser and rehydrator because of its high water content. Like all melons, cantaloupes are easiest to digest when they are the only food eaten at the meal, unless, of course, the other foods are other melons. Cantaloupe has lots of zinc, which is important for the prostate gland. Instead of the mid-morning or mid-afternoon snack of coffee or soda with a doughnut or cookie, eat half a cantaloupe. It makes a *great* snack and contains more vitamins A and C than an equal amount of just about any other fruit. It's also a powerhouse of potassium; a quarter of a cantaloupe offers between 800 to 900 mg. That's 25% of your daily potassium requirement! (For comparison, 1 cup lima beans has 950 mg; 1 cup tomato sauce has 900 mg; and 1 medium banana has about 450 mg.) According to new research, if you're not getting enough potassium, you could be putting yourself at risk for a stroke. Scientists tracked 5,600 adults for four to eight years and found that those who didn't eat enough potassium were 1.5 to 2.5 times more likely to suffer from a stroke, even if they were on medications to help prevent stroke.

I take cut-up cantaloupe pieces to snack on when I fly or drive in the car for hours. It also makes the perfect food to eat exclusively throughout the day (mono-diet) as a great once-a-month detoxifier and rejuvenator.

*See **Heavenly Cantaloupe Cocktail** recipe on page 113.*

Carrots

Coming in at 210 on the ORAC unit score for vegetables, carrots are a stellar detoxifier and an excellent food for the health of the liver and digestive tract. Naturally sweet, they make an ideal high-fiber, low-calorie snack food. Those baby carrots you find already peeled and packaged in your grocery store are not really baby carrots, but simply prepared to look that way.

You've all heard that old maxim about the benefits of carrots for your eyes. Well, there's some truth to that. Carrots contain a broad mix of carotenoids, including lutein and zeaxanthin, which help prevent cataracts, macular degeneration, and night blindness. In fact, it may be possible to delay the development of night-vision disturbances in later life by eating a wide variety of orange vegetables, especially carrots. These orange vegetables all contain vitamin A, and the more vitamin A you have in your body, the more rhodopsin you produce. Rhodopsin is a purple pigment that your eyes need in order to see in dim light. Carrots also contain additional antioxidants, including alpha-carotene, which fights cancer and heart disease. One of the reasons they are deemed as a heart-healthy food is because they are rich in calcium pectate, a soluble fiber that lowers cholesterol.

Carrots are one of those rare foods that increase in nutritional value when cooked (I still prefer them raw) because the heat breaks down the tough cellular walls that encase the beta-carotene, making it more available to us. To convert beta-carotene to vitamin A, the body needs at least a small amount of fat, because vitamin A is soluble in fat, not water. For that reason, I eat carrots with a little healthful fat such as avocado, nuts or seeds, or flax oil (often combined in a salad). Grated carrots hold an esteemed place of honor in most of my salads that are topped with a healthful dressing.

My friends all know when I've been juicing carrots to mix with my other green vegetables because my skin turns a faint shade of orange-yellow. A condition known as carotenosis, it is most common in children, but also appears in adults. It's harmless—so don't worry if you discover a color change in your skin. All you need to do is simply skip eating and juicing carrots for a few days, and your skin color will return to normal. Then you can begin enjoying them again, in a little more moderation.

As I've mentioned, eating primarily a whole-foods diet is best, but juicing can be a healthful addition to the program. "When a vegetable is fed into a juicing machine," writes Dr. George H. Malkmus in the spring 2005 issue of the quarterly magazine *Back to the Garden*, "the machine automatically separates the pulp and fiber from the juice; with the fiber removed, that raw vegetable juice we drink can go almost intravenously into the blood system, with approximately 92% of the nutrients reaching cellular level. Therefore, removing the fiber before we put the raw living food into our bodies takes a heavy load off the digestive system." He goes on to write: "So, when we juice, we not only satisfy our bodies' liquid needs, but also, because that freshly extracted vegetable juice is alive with enzymes and loaded with nutrients, we also satisfy the nutritional needs of our bodies simultaneously." (For more information on the informative, motivating magazine *Back to the Garden*, visit: **www.hacres.com**.)

See **Carotenoid Cocktail** recipe on page 113.

Celery

Celery can be traced back to the Greeks and Romans. In fact, they thought so highly of celery that they used it to crown the heads of distinguished guests. Low in calories and a good source of fiber and natural sodium, celery is also one of the world's greatest and most natural tranquilizers. It is an excellent tonic to soothe one's jangled nerves. (Maybe we should supply the leaders of all countries with a few stalks of celery every day!) Because of its calming effect on the central nervous system, celery makes a great night-time tonic for insomniacs. For that reason, a glass of celery-carrot juice is a good choice for a before-bedtime snack. Celery leaves are the most nutritious part of the plant, containing more calcium, iron, potassium, beta-carotene, and vitamin C than the stalks.

Let's dispel the erroneous rumor that celery is unhealthfully high in sodium. It's not! The form of sodium found in celery is organic and vital to all of the major organs. The noxious sodium is the table salt we add to foods, not the sodium we get in naturally balanced, sodium-rich organic foods. Celery leaves should be salvaged for soups, salads, and other dishes enhanced by the flavor of celery. I frequently juice several celery stalks and use this juice as a base for salad dressings, for vegetable smoothies (refer to my website: **www.SusanSmithJones.com** for more recipes), or to mix with other vegetable juices. Because it's rich in potassium, celery juice is also a perfect post-workout tonic. It replaces lost electrolytes, tones the vascular system, and lowers blood pressure.

Celery and celery seeds are our best dietary source of coumarins, a flavonoid compound with the potential to inhibit various forms of cancer. Studies have found that celery is also effective in helping prevent colon and stomach cancer; mollifying kidney and liver disorders; and easing gout, rheumatoid arthritis, and rheumatism. Celery juice taken before a meal curbs appetite and is, therefore, a natural diet aid.

See **Phytonutrient Power Drink** recipe on page 115.

Chili Peppers

A popular ingredient in Southwestern cooking, chilis (hot peppers) add spice and interest to many foods. I consume the milder varieties as low-calorie, nutritious snacks. Have you ever noticed that you feel so good after eating chilis that you want more? According to Dharma Singh Khalsa, MD, in his book *Food as Medicine,* that's because chilis raise your endorphin level. They're also bursting with a cornucopia of many nutrients, including impressive amounts of beta-carotene and vitamin C. In fact, chilis are so rich in vitamin C that they have been used as natural remedies for colds, coughs, bronchitis, and sinusitis around the globe. Just one raw, red hot pepper (1½ oz./45 grams) contains about 65 mg of vitamin C, nearly 100% of the RDA. Chilis also are rich in bioflavonoids, plant pigments that scientists believe help prevent cancer. Because chilis (red or green ones and jalapeños) have been found effective in lowering low-density lipoprotein (LDL), they act as preventive medicine against strokes, high blood pressure, and heart attacks. Research also indicates that the ingredient that makes chilis hot—capsaicin—may help prevent blood clots that can lead to a heart attack or stroke by acting as an anticoagulant. Capsaicinoids have been incorporated into topical creams and recommended to help alleviate the pain of arthritis by simply rubbing it on aching joints.

Remember, please, to handle chilis with care. When I'm preparing meals with them, I wear thin gloves, am careful not to rub my eyes, and always wash all utensils well with soap.

Cinnamon

Most people love the taste of cinnamon. Its fragrance conjures up thoughts of the holidays and special treats for the taste buds. An ancient spice obtained from the dried bark of two Asian evergreens, cinnamon is a highly versatile flavoring as well as a carminative that relieves bloating and gas.

Adding cinnamon to food, especially to sugary ones, helps normalize blood sugar by making insulin more sensitive. Cinnamon's most active ingredient is methylhydroxy chalcone polymer (MHCP), which increases the processing of blood sugar by 2,000%, or 20-fold. So using cinnamon in tiny amounts—even sprinkled in desserts—makes insulin more efficient. Cloves, turmeric, and bay leaves also work, but they're weaker. This is great news! Avoiding high circulating levels of blood sugar and insulin may help ward off diabetes and obesity. *Steady lower insulin levels are a sign of slower aging and greater longevity.*

Most days I find ways to include cinnamon in my meals. I sprinkle it on fruits and cereal; blend it in smoothies; and incorporate it in fruit sauces, purées, soups, and squash dishes. Don't forget to put cinnamon sticks in your tea or other hot beverages. I also make sachets of cinnamon, nutmeg, and cloves for gifts to hang in the kitchen, closets, linen cupboard, or laundry room.

See **Citrus Cinnamon Delight** recipe on page 121.

Coconut

Coconut butter (also referred to as coconut oil) has been used as a food and a medicine since the dawn of history. Ayurveda (the medicine of India) has long advocated its therapeutic and cosmetic properties. Unlike the cooked, clogging, cholesterol-laden, saturated fats found in meats and dairy products, coconut butter is a raw saturated fat containing mostly medium-chain fatty acids, which the body can metabolize efficiently and convert to energy quickly. Coconut butter contains no cholesterol and does not elevate "bad" (LDL) cholesterol levels. By weight, coconut butter has fewer calories than any other fat source. The medium-chain fatty acids (MCFAs) in coconut butter possess incredible properties. Bruce Fife, CN, ND, author of the terrific book *The Coconut Oil Miracle,* has written: "Coconut oil is, in essence, naturally antibacterial, antiviral, and antifungal." Added regularly to a balanced diet, it may help lower cholesterol by promoting its conversion into pregnenolone. Pregnenolone is the precursor to many hormones, including progesterone. Rich in magnesium, potassium, zinc, folate, and vitamin C, coconut also helps regulate thyroid function.

Coconut butter can be eaten straight or blended into a salad dressing, mixed into a smoothie, or incorporated into raw food cuisine. It also can be used as a skin lotion. It's very effective against dry skin and is ideal for massage. This is one of the main moisturizers I've used on my skin for years; I also use it on my hair as a biweekly deep conditioner. Coconut butter should be stored in a cool, dark area. Most butters and oils are light-sensitive, so make sure it is in a dark container to ensure that no light penetrates and causes damage. Always choose a raw, cold-pressed coconut butter, never heated. I also drink the delicious water from the young coconut. I often add the juice of half a small lemon to this water. It's a superb elixir and rejuvenating tonic for all ages. Additionally, I freeze the coconut water in ice-cube trays (in the shape of hearts, dolphins, stars, shells, lemons, and strawberries) along with a sprinkling of lemon zest in each cube. I put these frozen-coconut-water-with-lemon-zest cubes in glasses of water, tea, or other juice. Simply delicious and elegant!

See **Coconut Fruit Smoothie** recipe on page 118.

Cranberries

These tart red berries are not just for the holidays. Whole cranberries can also perk up spring and summer compotes, salads, sauces, and muffins. I frequently dry them in my dehydrator and add them to trail mix, cereals, and sandwiches, and grind the dried ones to sprinkle on soups and salads. I always keep frozen organic cranberries on hand to add to my smoothies or to eat by themselves for a snack on a hot summer day. But there's more to this distinctively firm berry than its pretty color.

Cranberries possess more phenols than red grapes, according to a study in the *Journal of Agricultural and Food Chemistry* in 2001. Phenols are plant chemicals (antioxidants) that lower oxidation of LDL cholesterol. Antioxidant levels in the blood of cranberry juice sippers rose by as much as 121% after three months of drinking the juice. In 2003, it was reported that a daily glass or two of this piquant beverage also can raise HDL ("good") cholesterol by about 10% (AM Chem Soc meeting, 3/03). That means about a 40% reduction in heart disease risk.

Cranberries also make it hard for bacteria to stick around—literally. Researchers believe that proanthocyanins in cranberries prevent the bacterium *E. coli* from attaching to bladder walls and causing urinary tract infections. The effect can last for ten hours after you drink 8 oz. of a cranberry-juice beverage that contains at least 27% juice, according to a study published in the *Journal of the American Medical Association (JAMA)* in 2002. Cranberry juice also prevents bacteria from adhering to teeth, as reported in a recent Israeli study. So stock up on those berry phytochemicals. They help you color yourself healthy.

See **Cranberry Grape Plunge** *recipe on page 117.*
See **Cranberry Pineapple Relish** *recipe on page 126.*

Cucumbers

You've probably said or heard someone say, "I'm as cool as a cucumber." There is truth to that expression. The cucumber contains over 90% water (more water than any other food except its relative, the watermelon). This water keeps its internal temperature several degrees cooler than the surrounding atmosphere. In fact, a cucumber is about 20 degrees cooler on the inside than the air outside is on a hot day. If you want to be cool, too, munch on a cucumber; it's a perfect thirst-quencher, an effective diuretic, and also relieves edema. I refer to cucumbers as "homeostatic food"—a term I coined to describe a food that tends to restore normal health because of its ability to cleanse and purify the blood and gradually alter the excretory process to restore normal body functions. Cucumbers contain a digestive enzyme, erepsin, that breaks down protein, cleanses the intestines, and helps expel intestinal parasites, especially tapeworms.

Low in calories, cucumbers offer a good source of fiber and a fair amount of vitamin C, potassium, folate, B-complex, and the amino acids methionine and tryptophan. The skin of the cucumber contains some vitamin A, so I encourage you to buy organic varieties or kirby cukes—the kind used for pickles—so you don't need to peel them. Unlike commercially grown varieties, organic cucumbers and kirby cukes are not sprayed with wax to retard spoilage. Another reason not to peel cukes is because you'll lose out on the high quantities of silica found in the skin. This beautifying mineral strengthens the connective tissue that basically keeps us from falling apart! Tendons, muscles, cartilage, bones, ligaments, and skin . . . they all love silica. It even adds elasticity to your skin and is great for the complexion. This is one reason cucumbers are often an ingredient in so many beauty creams. If you are treating eczema, psoriasis, splitting nails, hair loss, or acne, put cucumber on the top of your "must-have" list. Slices of cucumber placed on your eyes reduce swelling.

Cucumbers are a superb vegetable to juice, especially because of their high water content. Fresh cucumber juice reduces the high uric acid content that causes rheumatic ailments leading to inflammation or degeneration of joints, muscles, ligaments, or tendons. An excellent alkalizer, cucumber juice also helps normalize blood pressure and, because of its temperature-regulating properties, makes a great drink when you have a fever. When purchasing cucumbers, look for dark-skinned firm ones with no soft spots or wrinkles, preferably unwaxed. For maximum longevity, store them in a breathable produce bag and refrigerate to keep your cool cukes cool. (Like bell peppers, cucumbers actually are fruits.)

See **Savory Cucumber Fennel Salad** *recipe on page 120.*

Figs

A fruit worshipped throughout the ages, both dried and fresh, figs have been a popular delicacy in the Mediterranean area at least since biblical times. Pliny, the Roman writer (A.D. 52–113), said, "Figs are restorative. They increase the strength of young people, preserve the elderly in better health and make them look younger with fewer wrinkles." Sounds good to me!

Figs provide us with a medley of nutrients, including calcium, magnesium, potassium, iron, and fiber. While called a fruit by most people, figs are actually flower receptacles and bud like other fruit blossoms on the bare branches. Fresh figs are truly at their best just picked from the tree, but because fresh figs typically bruise easily and spoil rapidly, most are dried or canned. Although high in calories—260 calories in 5 pieces—dried figs are a highly nutritious snack food, contributing about ⅛ of the RDAs of calcium, iron, and magnesium, as well as 5 grams of fiber, more than 750 mg of potassium, and reasonable amounts of vitamin B6 and folate. Consuming figs with a citrus fruit or other sources of vitamin C will increase the absorption of their iron.

There are literally hundreds of fig varieties, but only about half a dozen are grown commercially in California—brought to this state by the Spanish missionary fathers who first planted them at the San Diego Mission in 1759. Fig trees were then planted at each succeeding mission, going north through California. The *Mission* fig, California's leading black fig, takes its name from this history. The popular *Calimyrna* fig, golden brown in color, is the Smyrna variety that was brought to California's San Joaquin Valley from Turkey in 1882, and was renamed "Calimyrna" in honor of its new homeland.

The following varieties are grown, dried, and packaged for the consumer. The Calimyrna fig, noted for its delicious nutlike flavor and tender, golden skin, is the popular favorite for eating out of hand. The *Kadota* fig, the American version of the original Italian Dattato, is thick-skinned and possesses a beautiful creamy amber color when ripe. Practically seedless, this fig is a favorite for canning and preserving, as well as drying. The *Adriatic* fig, transplanted from the Mediterranean, is the most prolific of all the varieties. The high-sugar content retained as the fruit dries to a golden shade makes this fig the prime choice for fig bars and pastes. My favorite is the Mission; I love its distinctive flavor. Its deep purple shade darkens to a rich black when dried, making this fig an aesthetic, as well as an edible, delight in all recipes. Figs are harvested ripe and are very perishable. Buy figs slightly firm that are heavy for their size. Store them on a plate lined with paper towels in the refrigerator for up to three days.

See **Fabulous Fig Sauce** *recipe on page 128.*

Flaxseed

Mahatma Gandhi once said, "Wherever flaxseeds become a regular food item among the people, there will be better health." I totally agree. Often referred to as "nutritional gold", flaxseed is one of the oldest known cultivated plants used not only for food, but also for making linen. It's a rich source of dietary fiber, protein, mucilage, phenolic compounds, and essential fatty acids—in particular, omega-3s. As well as playing a critical role in normal physiology, essential fatty acids are shown to be therapeutic and protect against heart disease, cancer, autoimmune diseases such as multiple sclerosis and rheumatoid arthritis, and many skin diseases.

In addition, flaxseeds are by far the leading dietary source of a class of compounds called *lignans,* which are phytoestrogens, or plant estrogens. Like the indole-3-carbinol in broccoli, lignans alter the balance of estrogens in the body, favoring the production of an estrogen metabolite that appears to protect against breast cancer. Nutritionist Joanne Slavin at the University of Minnesota conducted two studies—one in premenopausal women and one in postmenopausal women—and found that in both groups, the balance of estrogens shifted in a favorable direction when the women ate a couple of tablespoons of flaxseed each day.

Numerous other studies have uncovered the benefits of flaxseed to help alleviate constipation and bloating, eliminate toxic waste, strengthen the blood, reduce inflammation, accelerate fat loss, and reduce depression. The viscous nature of soluble fibers such as flaxseed mucilage is believed to slow down digestion and absorption of starch, resulting in lower levels of blood glucose, insulin, and other endocrine responses. In one study, blood glucose response was around 27% less for breakfast meals that included flax bread. Flaxseed consumption (50 grams per day for four weeks) by young, healthy adults and by the elderly has been shown to increase the number of bowel movements per week by about 30%.

You can purchase whole, cracked, or milled flaxseeds. The advantage to buying whole seeds is that the omega-3 fatty acids in them won't oxidize on your shelf, since the outer coating of the seeds shields the acids within. The drawback is that the human body is unable to digest the uncracked seeds, so you need to grind them in the coffee grinder before eating them. (I use my grinder only for seeds and nuts to ensure that there's no transfer of flavors.) I put some seeds in my smoothies in the morning and let my blender do the work. You also can sprinkle the ground seeds on your cereal in the morning, on your yogurt or salads, or add them to bread or muffin dough the next time you bake. You even can stir the ground meal into juice or water, or add a spoonful of flax-seed oil to your smoothies.

As wonderful as the flaxseed is, it's important not to consume more than 2 to 3 tablespoons per day because the husks contain compounds that can be toxic in high doses.

Garlic

A versatile culinary NATUREFOOD with an ORAC score of 1,939, garlic has been around for ages. Herbalists and folk healers have used garlic to treat myriad diseases for thousands of years, and it has been intensively studied in recent years with hundreds of scientific papers published in medical journals since the mid-1980s. The ancient Greek physician Dioscorides reported that garlic could "clear the arteries", and Hippocrates prescribed it for intestinal disorders. In 1858, Louis Pasteur discovered that garlic could kill bacteria. And because Russian physicians used the garlic bulb to cure infections, it was known as "Russian penicillin" well into the 20th century. Albert Schweitzer is said to have used garlic as a cure for amoebic dysentery when he was in Africa.

Its therapeutic marvels aside, garlic is scrumptious to use in food preparations, and I always have several bulbs planted in my herb garden so I have fresh garlic greens to use. It's also a veritable treasure chest of nutrients. Garlic is a rich source of unique sulfur compounds that keep your body chemistry in balance. Similar compounds to those found in onions, leeks, and chives, they are thought to be responsible for garlic's antibacterial and antifungal activities, as well as its ability to slow cholesterol synthesis, lower blood pressure, reduce atherosclerosis, and inhibit platelet aggregation. The sulfur compounds even may prove to fight cancer. In the Iowa Women's Health Study, women who ate garlic at least once per week had a 32% lower risk of colon cancer than those who ate none. Research at the National Cancer Institute is showing that garlic extracts can both slow the proliferation of cancer cells and cause abnormal cells to self-destruct. (I've taken Kyolic Aged Garlic Extract for over 35 years.)

In European studies, garlic has been shown to help eliminate lead and other heavy metals from the body. It also is effective in removing worms and other parasites from the alimentary canal, boosting immune function, and improving the action of the liver and the gallbladder. To ward off mosquitoes, eat garlic once each day. For athlete's foot, spread crushed garlic once daily over the affected area (which will feel warm for about ten minutes) for a half hour before washing with water. If the crushed garlic "burns" your skin, wash immediately with cool water and repeat the next day with less garlic. Alternatively, you can sprinkle garlic powder daily on your wet feet and let dry before putting on your socks. (Visit: **www.kyolic.com.**)

Raw garlic has a sharp, biting flavor that some people find too strong for their taste. Cooking eliminates the bite (and squashes the flavor somewhat), and roasted garlic has a mild nutty flavor. Roast unpeeled cloves for 40-45 minutes at 350°; then peel; mash; and use in purées, sauces, and dressings.

Ginger

Fresh ginger tastes decidedly different from powdered ginger. The beige, knobby root has a bite, a sweetness, and a woodsy aroma all its own and is available year-round. Cut off as much ginger as needed. Gently peel the thin beige skin from the root. The flesh beneath the skin is the most flavorful. Slice the ginger into "coins". Slices will lend an indirect flavor to a variety of dishes. Unpeeled ginger, tightly wrapped, can be kept in the refrigerator for about three weeks. I juice it; drink it as a tea; chop it for sautés; and mince it for dips, sauces, soups, and purées. Minced ginger will give a more pungent flavor. Look for robust roots with a spicy fragrance. Signs of cracking or withering indicate old age.

Research is just beginning to confirm the centuries-old notion that ginger is health-promoting. It contains several antioxidant plant chemicals, including gingerol, shogaol, and zingerone. These antioxidants help fight cancer and heart disease. For example, water spiked with ginger extract, when given to mice, significantly slowed the development of mammary tumors, according to a Japanese study published in 2002. Ginger extract lowered total cholesterol (and LDL cholesterol too) and triglyceride levels and reduced atherosclerosis in mice, as revealed in a 2000 Israeli study. And gingerol is as effective as aspirin in preventing blood clotting. It thins the blood "just like aspirin", making it a potential aid against heart disease.

Ginger also promotes digestion, aids in nausea (great for motion sickness and morning sickness), and is a powerful anti-inflammatory. Inflammation is a suspect in heart disease, stroke, cancer, Alzheimer's disease, and arthritis. Gingerols reduce pain in animals and act as Cox-2 inhibitors, similar to the doctor-prescribed anti-arthritis drugs now available. University of Miami research shows that patients with osteoarthritis of the knee who took 255 mg of ginger extract twice each day for six weeks had less knee pain than those not getting ginger. So spice up your health and life with versatile ginger root.

Goji Berries

ometimes referred to as *wolfberries* or *lycium*, these bright orange-red berries are one of the most nutritionally dense fruits on the planet. About the size of a raisin, the goji berry has been heralded as a major anti-aging herb/fruit since the dawn of Asian civilization. Today, it is also one of the most popular fruits in Asia, rivaling foods like ginseng and reishi mushroom, widely revered as a superior health tonic.

Goji berries traditionally have been regarded as a longevity, strength-building, beautifying, and sexual-potency food of the highest order. In several study groups with elderly people in Asia, these berries were given once each day for three weeks, and 67% of the patients' T-cell transformation functions tripled, and the activity of the patients' white-cell interleukin-2 doubled. In addition, the results showed that all the patients' spirits and optimism increased significantly, 95% had improved appetite, 95% slept better, and 35% of the patients partially recovered their sexual function.

It is generally believed in Asia that those who consume goji berries over an extended period of time will have softer, blemish-free, wrinkle-resistant, youthful skin. Chinese martial-arts practitioners and athletes have been using these berries for over 2,000 years to strengthen their legs and promote endurance. The famed Li Qing Yuen, who was said to live to the age of 252 years (1678–1930), consumed several ounces of goji berries every day throughout his long life. The life of Li Qing Yuen is the best documented case of extreme longevity known.

These delicious berries contain 18 amino acids (six times higher than bee pollen), including all 8 essential amino acids (such as isoleucine and tryptophan). They also boast 21 trace minerals—the main ones being zinc, iron, copper, calcium, germanium, selenium, and phosphorus. But where they really shine is in their carotenoid content; they are the richest source of beta-carotene of all known foods on Earth! Goji berries also contain 500 times more vitamin C by weight than oranges, making them second only to camu camu berries as the world's richest source of vitamin C. They're also abounding with vitamins B_1, B_2, B_6, and vitamin E.

The best source of these beautiful berries is in protected valleys in million-year-old soil in remote cultivated areas of inner Mongolia and Tibet. The plants grow like bushes with vines that reach over 15 feet. The fresh berries are never touched by hand because, if they were, they would oxidize and turn black. Instead, they are shaken onto mats, then dried in the shade.

This colorful fruit tastes like a cross between a cranberry and a cherry. Goji berries make a tasty snack for adults and kids alike. Eat them by themselves or combine with other fruit, nuts, and seeds in a trail mix. Sprinkle them on salads, add to smoothies or fruit sauces, commingle them when baking in cookies and fruit pies, or soak them in warm water for ten minutes and mix them into oatmeal and pancakes. Drink the soaking liquid. Yum! Traditionally, it is believed that eating 1–2 oz. of fresh-dried goji berries per day will provide all of the benefits I've described. Ask for them at your local health-food store, grocery store, or farmers' market.

Grapefruit

As with all other citrus fruits, grapefruit is rich in vitamin C and potassium and very low in calories. A cup of freshly squeezed grapefruit juice has 95 mg of vitamin C, more than 100% of the adult RDA. This fresh, raw juice eases constipation and improves digestion by increasing the flow of gastric juices. One whole grapefruit has only 100 calories, and it makes a perfect snack food. The red and pink varieties are high in beta-carotene and lycopene.

Deep inside the white rind and membranes of this fruit (lemons and oranges too) lies a miraculous group of plant compounds—bioflavonoids, citric acids, and pectins. These plant compounds protect against cancer and heart disease. Grapefruit pectin reduces the accumulation of atherosclerotic plaque in patients afflicted with atherosclerosis and strengthens blood vessels and capillaries.

In *Foods That Harm, Foods That Heal* by Reader's Digest, I learned that some people with rheumatoid arthritis, lupus, and other inflammatory disorders find that eating grapefruit daily seems to alleviate their symptoms. This may occur because plant chemicals block the prostaglandins that cause inflammation.

Do you need to lose weight? Make grapefruit your first course to help prevent overeating. The pectin content of grapefruit reduces appetite by slowing the emptying of the stomach. In the battle against colds, grapefruit juice helps reduce fever and soothes coughs and sore throats. If I ever feel a cold coming on, which is rare, I blend one peeled grapefruit with some water, fresh ginger, and cayenne pepper, drink the liquid, and feel it work in minutes. A pinch of cinnamon is a tasty, healthful addition too. Consumed at night, grapefruit juice promotes sleep and alleviates insomnia. Adding the juice of half a lemon to your grapefruit drinks will cause excess mucus in your body to be dissolved. Think pink. Pink and red varieties are far more nutritious than white grapefruit.

See **Glorious Grapefruit Juice/Smoothie** recipe on page 117.

Green Leafy Vegetables

Green and leafy vegetables should become an essential part of your daily diet. They provide a treasure trove of vitamins and minerals needed for a healthy immune system. They also help ward off diseases such as cancer. Leafy greens are excellent for the gallbladder, spleen, heart, and blood, and are a good brain food and natural laxative. Most greens can be cooked or eaten raw in salads or fresh juices.

To clean them, use a natural produce cleaner or soak in a sink of cold water and the juice of one lemon for a few minutes and swirl around, then drain the water. Pat or spin dry. Tear the leaves into small pieces, trim the ends of the stems, and chop when necessary. All leafy greens contain chlorophyll, iron, magnesium, calcium, manganese, vitamin C, potassium, vitamin A, and a bonus of the essential fatty acids, with no cholesterol. The vegetables with the darkest, most intense colors tend to contain the highest level of nutrients. All lettuce is said to calm the nerves. Here is a brief listing of some of my favorite leafy greens I eat on a regular basis: arugula, beet greens, Belgian endive, butterhead lettuce, chicory, collards, dandelion greens, escarole and endive, kale, mustard and turnip greens, parsley, romaine lettuce, sorrel, spinach, Swiss chard, and watercress.

- *Arugula:* This green from the mustard family is peppery and tart and mixes well with other greens. It is also known as roquette. It adds pizzazz to any raw salad, is high in vitamins A and C, niacin, iron, and phosphorus, and is good for normalizing body acid with its high alkalinity.

- *Beet Greens:* Best used in juices, they are very high in nutrients, especially potassium, iron, and calcium. These greens also can be used in cooking. They are known for their benefit in blood disorders, liver function, and the flow of bile.

- *Belgian Endive:* Here's a delicious green that's great in a salad combined with avocado cubes and a light vinaigrette dressing; I also use the leaves for dipping in place of crackers or chips. Make a pinwheel design on a plate with the leaves and stuff them with chopped vegetables or hummus. It has pale yellow or white leaves and is similar to chicory in healing qualities and nutrient content.

- *Butterhead Lettuce:* Also known as Boston Bibb, this is a very tender leaf, with an almost buttery taste. It makes a good salad when used alone or with spinach, endive, or watercress.

- *Chicory:* This is a bitter green with curly leaves; the young leaves are best in salads. It's high in vitamins A and C, calcium, and iron, and aids in liver function and blood disorders. Try radicchio, often called red-leaf chicory, which is great in salads and adds a stunning, beautiful color.

- *Collards:* This brilliant green vegetable is a member of the cabbage family. Use only the leaves. They tend to be tough, so you may want to steam them for a few minutes. Collards can be used in salads as a substitute for cabbage and are also great for juicing. Because of its high nutrient content, no leafy green is more valuable in the body for disorders of the colon, respiratory system, lymphatic system, and skeletal system.

- *Dandelion Greens:* The young leaves have a tangy taste. They are good for gallbladder disorders, rheumatism, gout, eczema, and skin disorders. Dandelion is also an excellent liver rejuvenator. They cook the same as any leafy green. They are rich in calcium, potassium, and vitamins A and C. These are also excellent to add to juices.

- *Escarole and Endive:* From the chicory family, the leaves are very dark green, with a slightly bitter taste. These make a good salad (with a citrus-flavored dressing) and also can be steamed. Both are rich in vitamin A, B-vitamins, and minerals such as calcium, potassium, and iron. They're good for most infections, liver function, and internal cleansing.

- *Kale:* This is the king of calcium. Use only the leaves of this plant unless juicing. It tastes like cabbage. I often add the juice of kale to carrot and other fresh vegetable juices. It's very high in usable calcium and is excellent for prevention and care of osteoporosis.

- *Mustard and Turnip:* These greens have a zippy taste with flavors varying from mild to hot. They are good sautéed with a little garlic or steamed, and also can be used in juices. They are high in calcium and vitamin C and are good for infections, colon disorders, colds, flu, and elimination of kidney stones due to excess uric acid.

- *Parsley:* All types of this green herb are rich in vitamins A, B-complex, and C, and minerals such as potassium and manganese. Parsley contains mucilage, starch, opinol, and volatile oil. It is very crisp and tangy. This green has an "odor-eating" quality that helps restore fresh breath after a meal with such foods as garlic and onion. Add curly or flat-leaf parsley to fresh juice or chop to add to salads. It's good for digestive disorders and also an excellent diuretic. Also try cilantro, a Chinese and Mexican parsley, essential in many Chinese, Spanish, Mexican, and Thai dishes.

- *Romaine Lettuce:* This is my favorite lettuce green. It's a wonderful, crunchy green that is highest in nutrients of all types of lettuce, including rich amounts of vitamins C and K and carotenoids. It's great in salads. I always keep lots on hand for salads and juicing and usually go through one head each day just for myself. Romaine is not recommended for cooking. Being high in chlorophyll, it's a good blood purifier.

- *Sorrel:* This green has a pleasantly sour and slightly lemon flavor. It's easily perishable and best bought fresh or grown in your garden. Try sorrel in salads or as a seasoning in soups and casseroles. Sorrel is a powerful antioxidant with the same healing properties as kale.

- *Spinach:* Its tender, bright green leaves are most beneficial when eaten raw. Because of the oxalic acid content, some of the calcium becomes unavailable to the body. Spinach contains many valuable nutrients and is high in chlorophyll, potassium, and iron.

- *Swiss Chard:* From the beet family, this green has a mild taste and is good with walnuts or pine nuts added to a salad. It has the highest content of sodium of all greens. Chlorophyll- and calcium-rich, Swiss chard is a natural cleanser and helps strengthen bones. Look for Swiss chard in red, green, and rainbow colors.

- *Watercress:* This green has young, tender leaves that should be picked before the plant flowers. The spicy-flavored green goes well with romaine and butterhead lettuce. It's higher in nutrient content than most greens and is excellent for vitamin deficiencies and illnesses of all types. It's good added to fresh juices too.

Experiment with your salads and fresh vegetable juices; and mix and match these greens to make a variety of delicious, nutritious dishes and drinks.

Kale

As recommended earlier, kale is one of the most nutritious greens in the garden. It's part of the cruciferous family and is a rich source of indoles, glucosinolates, and isothiocyanates, a group of potent phytochemicals that help prevent breast and lung cancers. The high content of the carotenoids lutein and zeaxanthin in kale helps prevent age-related macular degeneration of the eyes. As a rich source of chlorophyll, this vegetable oxygenates the blood, improves red-blood-cell counts, and aids the fundamental processes of cell circulation and respiration. As if that weren't enough, kale also is an outstanding source of beta-carotene, vitamins C and E, and calcium. In fact, a cup of kale surpasses the calcium content found in a glass of milk and, because it contains an unusually high ratio of calcium to phosphorus, the calcium found in kale is absorbed far more successfully. Adding to these accolades, kale is also rich in folate, iron, zinc, potassium, and magnesium.

Few vegetables compare to kale when it comes to its nutritional beauty. The best way to feed your trillions of cells with this God-given treasure is by juicing it. Combine kale with other green vegetables and herbs (such as celery, Swiss chard, collard greens, romaine lettuce, mustard greens, watercress, dandelion, arugala, cucumber, parsley, or beet tops or any combination thereof) and some carrot and/or apple for sweetener. On an empty stomach, this super tonic will revitalize your cells and body in minutes.

* * *

III

INTERMISSION

HEALING POWER OF RAW FOODS & FRESH JUICES

"Out of clutter, find simplicity. From discord, find harmony.
In the middle of difficulty, lies opportunity."

—Albert Einstein

Scientists and doctors are now emphasizing the importance of fresh, raw foods in our diet due to the loss of essential vitamins, enzymes, friendly bacteria, and other food factors caused by cooking. Modern scientific medicine is finally catching up with traditional wisdom and helping us prevent the diseases caused by the Standard American Diet (appropriately known as the "SAD" diet).

The core philosophy of the raw-food movement revolves around the idea that enzymes, the catalysts needed to aid digestion and nutrient absorption, are destroyed at temperatures around 118°F (some say 108°F). Without these food enzymes, our bodies have to work harder to digest and assimilate the foods we consume. Enzyme-rich foods help provide our bodies with a more viable and efficient energy source. Raw foods rapidly digest in our stomach and begin to provide energy and nutrition at a quick rate.

Consuming cooked food, either alone or before raw food, can cause a condition called leukocytosis, an increase in white blood cells. Your body may respond to cooked food as if it were a foreign bacterium or a diseased cell, which causes your immune system to waste energy on defending you. By eating only raw food or eating raw food prior to eating cooked food, you can prevent leukocytosis.

While the body also produces enzymes, some researchers believe that only finite amounts of them are available over the course of a lifetime. They theorize that as the enzyme supply dwindles, the body ages more quickly, has less ability to fight disease, and essentially runs out of energy. Because raw food is in its original, natural form, it is more wholesome, assimilative, and digestible. Food eaten raw puts very little stress on the body's systems. Gabriel Cousens, MD, recommends raw foods for many reasons, including their alkalinity, their high enzyme levels, and their ability to improve circulation. He says, "Live-cell-analysis experimentation has shown that within ten minutes after ingesting enzymes, red blood cells become unclumped. Something is happening in the blood after the enzymes are ingested that suggests the enzymes are effective in the blood." In other words, the live enzymes in raw foods have a healing effect on the body.

In her delightful book, *Angel Foods: Healthy Recipes for Heavenly Bodies,* Cherie Soria writes that food, like all matter, is vibrational energy. When we consume it, the vibration of the food is transferred to us as vital life force. Therefore, the more fresh and alive the food, the more life force we receive. This life force can be observed using Kirlian photography, and according to Soria, "Double-blind studies have proven that awareness of this life force strengthens and magnifies the subtle energy even more." When volunteers in scientific experiments directed their healing energy into water, and the water was then given to plants, the plants grew faster, larger, and more resistant to disease! Soria encourages us to do the same thing with our foods by focusing love energy into them as we prepare our meals. I have always loved preparing foods, but now I consciously bring my connection with nature and the Divine into the kitchen with me.

I find that raw food provides a far greater range of taste than cooked food. The most popular misconception is that raw food is all one texture: crunch. Matthew Kenney and Sarma Melngailis, head chefs and co-owners of the popular New York City raw food restaurant Pure Food and Wine, have dispelled this notion in their resplendent book, *Raw Food/Real World: 100 Recipes to Get the Glow,* which takes raw foods to a sublimely gourmet level. The lushly colorful pages illustrate the authors' magic—vividly showing that preparing and eating raw food can be an exquisite delight (and not at all time-consuming). You'll learn that there is a whole range of textures, such as creamy and chewy. Raw foods can be served warm, cold, or just cool, and the right spices add heat and excitement.

CHANGE YOUR DIET, CHANGE YOUR LIFE

I've emphasized raw foods for years and teach courses in "Living Food Cuisine". Participants new to this way of eating and living—it's more a lifestyle than just a "diet"—are always astounded by how great they feel after a few days on raw foods. "We have seen tremendous positive changes in our health, as well as witnessed many health benefits in others who eat a predominantly raw food diet," write Charles Nungesser and George Nungesser in their book, *How We All Went RAW: Raw Food Recipe Book.* "We have seen major turnarounds in cancer, heart disease, diabetes, hypoglycemia, thyroid disorders, hormone imbalance, weight problems, and many other health struggles. After seeing all these benefits, we were convinced there is *something powerful* to raw foods."

PERSONAL CHANGES

The changes I've seen when eating more raw foods go beyond physical to the mental, emotional, and spiritual. I experience more inner peace, joy, harmony, and clarity. My eyes become clearer and more violet-blue, any extra weight falls away, my skin becomes softer, wrinkles abate, and people tell me that I look younger. I have more energy throughout the day, feel a deeper connection with my own Divinity, and feel a greater sense of connectedness with all life. That's why I often refer to it as *spiritual* nutrition. Try it for 30 days and you'll see a big difference in your life. It's hard to put into words the feeling of balance, well-being, and personal power you experience when eating a raw-food diet.

Elisabetta Politi, the head of nutrition at Duke University Diet & Fitness Center, says that any way of eating that promotes minimal food processing needs to be considered seriously. "I think people would benefit from having more raw foods in a well-balanced diet," she says, while cautioning that an entirely raw diet would be very difficult to sustain for most of the population.

I am the first to admit that eating 100% raw is not an easy thing to do when you need to integrate into "normal" society. And I also don't suggest that you switch to all raw foods overnight. In my books and workshops, I recommend beginning with adding 50% raw food to each meal. For example, you might add a juice or a smoothie with breakfast or add in a generous portion of fresh fruit to your cereal. For lunch, include a garden salad and a different salad at dinner, along with some cooked food. For your snacks, try some fresh fruit, vegetable juice, cut-up raw vegetables, healthy trail mix, or some raw-fruit pudding or raw-vegetable soup. (See my website for recipes: **www.SusanSmithJones.com.**)

ADJUSTING YOUR LIFESTYLE FOR HEALTHIER CHOICES

Before eating cooked food, always start with a few bites of raw food. Or upgrade the 50% raw regimen to include two days a week with raw meals. For example, on Monday you eat only raw foods until dinner, giving you 24 hours on raw food (since Sunday dinner). On Thursday, eat raw foods at all of your meals, giving you 36 hours on raw food (from Wednesday dinner to Friday breakfast). Weekdays seem to be easier than weekends for most of my clients.

If you have no desire to eat a totally raw-food diet, I encourage you to aspire to at least 60%, or better yet, 75–85% raw foods. From my experience, having worked with thousands of people, it seems that this higher amount of raw food versus cooked food will make a profound difference in how you feel and look. I am not a "raw-food purist". I still enjoy cooking and going out to eat, but most of the time I consume healthful raw foods. Remember, raw doesn't necessarily mean cold. Foods may be warmed to well above body temperature and still maintain their life force. A good rule of thumb is: if you stick your finger in it, it should feel warm—not hot. In order to create many of the foods in a raw-food diet, or simply make healthful cooked meals easily without spending hours in the kitchen, it's helpful to have a few beneficial tools. (See page 134.)

ALKALIZE & ENERGIZE

In his popular book, *Alkalize or Die,* author and friend Dr. Theodore A. Baroody writes about the importance of living a lifestyle that supports alkalinity. When foods are eaten, they are broken down into small components and delivered to each and every cell in the body. These nutrients are burned with oxygen in a slow, controlled manner to supply the necessary energy for us to function. After oxidation, the cells excrete waste products.

The digestion of foods—*all* foods, healthful or unhealthful—results in waste products. The difference between healthful food and unhealthful food is the amount and kind of wastes produced: acid or alkaline. Human cells die in about four weeks; some regenerate and some are destroyed. Dead cells are waste products. All waste products need to be discarded from the body, mostly through urine and perspiration. Most of these wastes are acidic; therefore, when we excrete them, our urine is acidic and our skin is acidic.

Most of us overwork, stay up late, get up early, and stress ourselves to the limit without giving ourselves time to rest. Most people like to eat meat and refined grains and enjoy colas and other soft drinks, which are all highly acidic foods and drinks. Furthermore, the polluted environment kills our healthy cells, thus producing more acidic wastes. This means that we cannot get rid of 100% of the acidic wastes that we make daily, and these leftover wastes are stored somewhere within our bodies.

Since our blood and cellular fluids must be slightly alkaline to sustain life, the body converts liquid acidic wastes into solid wastes. Solidification of liquid acid wastes is the body's defense mechanism to survive. Some of these acid wastes include cholesterol, fatty acid, uric acid, kidney stones, phosphates, sulfates, urates, and gallstones; and they accumulate in many places throughout our body. (For 15 years, I've used AlkaLife® drops. Visit: **www.alkalife.com.**)

One of the biggest problems caused by the build-up of acidic wastes is the fact that *acid coagulates blood.* When blood becomes thicker, it clogs up the capillaries, which is why so many adult diseases require blood thinners as part of their treatment. It is commonly known that degenerative diseases are caused by poor blood circulation. Where there is an accumulation of acidic wastes, and the local capillaries are clogged, any organ(s) in that area will be deprived of an adequate blood supply, which can eventually lead to dysfunction of that organ or those organs.

Doctors have found that more than 150 degenerative diseases are associated with acidity, including cancer, diabetes, arthritis, heart disease, and gall and kidney stones. All diseases thrive in an acidic, oxygen-poor environment.

The symbol "pH" (power of hydrogen) is a measurement of how acidic or alkaline a substance is. The pH scale goes from 1 to 14. For example, a reading of 1pH would be acidic, a reading of 7pH would be neutral, and a reading of 14pH would be alkaline.

Keep in mind that a drop in every point on the pH scale is 10 times more acid (that is, from 7 to 6 is 10 times, from 7 to 5 is 100 times, etc.). From 7 to 2 is 100,000 times more acidic! And sodas are in the acidic range of 2 pH. Over the long term, the effects of sodas are devastating to the body. Acidity, sugars, and artificial sweeteners can shorten your life. In fact, *it takes 32 glasses of alkaline water at a pH of 9 to neutralize the acid from one can of cola or soda.* When you drink sodas, the body uses up reserves of its own stored alkaline buffers—mainly calcium from the bones and DNA—to raise the body's alkalinity levels, especially to maintain proper blood-alkaline pH levels. Acidic blood levels can cause death!

If you want to know your current acid-alkaline balance, you can check your pH with a simple saliva test by using litmus paper that comes with a color chart. To properly check your saliva pH, bring up your saliva twice and spit it out. Bring it up a third time, but don't spit it out. Put the litmus strip under your tongue and wet it with your saliva. To find your pH level, match the color of the litmus strip to the corresponding color on the chart. Your goal is to have an alkaline (7.1–7.5) pH level. Note that it is natural for you to be more alkaline in the morning and more acidic at night.

Most of the degenerative diseases that we call "old-age diseases", like memory loss, osteoporosis, arthritis, diabetes, and hypertension, are actually lifestyle diseases caused by acidosis, an overall poor diet (especially a lack of leafy green vegetables), improper digestion, and too much stress.

So how can you alkalize your body? Baroody suggests following an 80%/20% dietary rule. Choose 80% alkaline-forming foods and drinks and 20% acid-forming foods and drinks for vibrant health. In *Alkalize or Die,* he groups foods into categories, based on whether they are acid, alkaline, or neutral. In a nutshell, most fruits and vegetables are alkaline and most other foods, including meat, dairy, fish, fowl, grains, seeds, and nuts are acid-forming. He recommends that we build up to eating a diet of 75% fresh and raw plant-based foods and 25% cooked foods. He encourages the daily practice of meditation, deep breathing, exercise, deep sleep, and positive thinking—all of which increase alkalinity.

One of the quickest and best ways to improve health and increase alkalinity is to make fresh vegetable juice every day. Chlorophyll, which gives green vegetables their color, builds the blood and powerfully alkalizes the system. Now, let's explore the benefits of juicing.

JUICING FOR RADIANT HEALTH & VITALITY

Countless studies show that a high intake of fresh fruits and vegetables can lower the incidence of heart problems, cancer, and the degenerative diseases of aging. The evidence is so convincing, in fact, that the U.S. recommended daily allowance of fruits and vegetables has increased. Additionally, the more colorful and natural your diet—especially nutrient- and antioxidant-rich produce—the healthier and more youthful you'll become.

One way to increase your daily consumption of fresh fruits and vegetables is through juicing. Freshly made juices are concentrated nutritional elixirs that heal and rejuvenate the body and help bring balance to all the body's cells. Juicing is also one of the easiest, most efficient, and most delicious ways to ensure you are meeting your daily produce quota.

Juicing is different from blending. When you juice, you separate the juice of the fruit or vegetable from the fiber. You are probably thinking, *Why would I do that? Fiber is essential for good health.* I agree and recommend both a high-fiber diet *and* fresh vegetable juices. The fiber found in raw vegetables, fresh fruits, and other plant-based foods (animal products don't have any fiber) plays a vital role in the health of the colon, the promotion of regular bowel movements, and the transport of toxins out of the body. To maximize the benefits of a whole-foods diet, we need a good balance of and an emphasis on whole raw foods, as close to the way nature made them as possible, as well as freshly extracted raw-vegetable juices. To understand more clearly, here is a nutshell view of digestion.

Digestion begins in the mouth. As you chew your food, it is mixed with your salivary enzymes before it moves on to your stomach and intestines. Ultimately, the food is liquefied so that the nutrients can pass from the small intestine into the bloodstream and lymph fluid for distribution. The remaining fiber is passed into the colon for elimination after excess water and remaining minerals are absorbed. Since its fiber is already removed, fresh juice provides a treasure chest of pure nutrients that require little digestive effort for optimal utilization.

MAXIMIZING YOUR NUTRIENT INTAKE

Unless you take steps to counteract the dietary trends of modern society, you will be overfed (though likely malnourished because of low-nutrient foods) and burdened with a heavy load of internal toxicity. Your body is designed to be self-healing, self-renewing, and self-rejuvenating, but it only can accomplish that if you give it the right ingredients, including nutrients from raw, living foods. Juicing is an easy and effective way to maximize your nutrient intake without putting a heavy digestive burden on your body. It also helps the body eliminate toxins.

In *The Juicing Book,* by Stephen Blauer, I found this passage by the late Bernard Jensen, PhD. "By adding fresh juices to a balanced food regimen, you will help accelerate and enhance the process of restoring nutrients to chemically starved tissues. It is on these tissues that disease and illness thrive. In terms of prevention, therefore, the importance of juices cannot be overstated."

In *Live Food Juices,* H. E. Kirschner, MD, says that if modern research is correct, the power to break down the cellular structure of raw vegetables and assimilate the precious elements they contain is only fractional (35% in the healthiest individuals, as low as 1% in the less healthy). But, he adds, when drinking juices, these same individuals assimilate up to 92% of these elements. Blauer concurs: "Fresh juice is more than an excellent source of vitamins, minerals, enzymes, purified water, proteins, carbohydrates, and chlorophyll. Because it is in liquid form, fresh juice supplies nutrition that is not wasted to fuel its own digestion as it is with whole fruits, vegetables, and grasses. As a result, the body can quickly and easily make maximum use of all the nutrition that fresh juice offers."

Because of the high sugar content of modern hybridized fruit (organic fruits, too), I generally advocate eating whole fruit and juicing vegetables. In addition to making fresh vegetable juice every day, I do an exclusive day of juice fasting once every two weeks and 2–3 consecutive days a month, consuming nothing but fresh vegetable juices, water, and my favorite teas. It's easy, fun, and provides the stamina I need to engage in my daily activities without necessitating much alteration of lifestyle. You just need a high-quality juicer.

It takes a pound of carrots to make about 10 oz. of carrot juice. Could you eat that many carrots? Probably not. Yet all the enzymes, water soluble vitamins, minerals, phytonutrients, and trace elements in those carrots are extracted and condensed into the glass of juice. The same thing applies to other vegetables. You might have a hard time eating 4–7 servings of vegetables each day, but it's easy to consume the nutritional value of a variety of vegetables by juicing them.

In light of all of the research on the benefits of fresh vegetable juices, it's difficult to understand why anyone would not favor the addition of fresh vegetable juices to their diet. Michael Donaldson, PhD, head of the Hallelujah Acres Foundation, conducted a study to determine the effect of carrot juice on blood-glucose levels. He found, contrary to popular thinking, that the body actually handles the raw carrot juice very efficiently, with much less impact on the blood glucose than eating whole-grain bread. You can review the study at **www.hacres.com**. For people with blood-sugar issues, adding a teaspoon of fresh flaxseed oil or ground flaxseed meal to the juice can further lower the glucose response to carrot juice.

Another option is to make the juice a combination of 50% carrot and 50% green leafy lettuce or other dark green vegetables. Here are just a few of the vegetables I juice: spinach, celery, beets, cucumbers, romaine lettuce, Swiss chard, kale, collards, cauliflower, green onions, mustard greens, broccoli and brussels sprouts, bell peppers, cabbage, and carrots. I also sometimes add parsley, lemon, apple, tomato, garlic, and ginger. You'll find a variety of juicing recipes in this book and on my audio programs, which are available from my website.

FRESH JUICE IS THE BEST

You can find juices at your local natural food store, but it's always best to make them fresh. As a culinary instructor, whole-foods chef, and a holistic health coach for over 30 years, one of my passions is helping my clients and friends create healthy kitchens. For starters, I always encourage purchasing a top-quality juicer. The one I use and recommend is the Champion 2000+ Juicer. (See page 137 for more details and ordering information.) When using a Champion, the preparation of fresh, wholesome fruit and vegetable juices of the highest quality couldn't be easier.

* * *

IV

MORE ENTRÉES

50 NATUREFOODS

Part II

Now, let's continue with our perusal of the 50 revitalizing NATUREFOODS that will help you along on the path to better health, wellness, and vitality, qualities that can greatly enhance your self-esteem and enjoyment of life.

Remember, while I am singing the praises of these best-of-the-best foods and describing their extraordinary health benefits, keep in mind that *all* fresh fruits, vegetables, legumes, raw nuts and seeds, and whole grains bring tremendous benefits. The unsurpassed nutrients and other qualities I describe for individual foods are also found to varying degrees in *all* of the NATUREFOODS I recommend for a complete, overall healthful diet.

Kiwi

One of the most underrated of all fruits, kiwi has an ORAC score of 602 for 3½ oz., higher than all fruits except cherries (670), grapes (739), oranges (750), avocados (782), plums (949), raspberries (1,220), strawberries (1,540), cranberries (1,750), blackberries (2,036), blueberries (2,400), raisins (2,830), and prunes (5,770). This egg-shaped fruit with a fuzzy brown skin originated in China and was known as the Chinese gooseberry until New Zealand fruit growers renamed it for their national bird and began exporting it. Once considered an exotic fruit, kiwis now are grown in California and have become increasingly plentiful. They are harvested while green and can be kept in cold storage for six to ten months, making them available for most of the year.

Not only are kiwis high in vitamin C, containing 16 times more than oranges, they also contain an impressive amount of vitamin E. The kiwi's bright green flesh, which is dotted with tiny, edible black seeds, provides a good amount of the mineral potassium as well as pectin, a soluble fiber that helps control blood-cholesterol levels. Each 3 oz. serving has only 56 calories and provides 85 mg of vitamin C. Kiwis also contain both lutein and zeaxanthin, antioxidants associated with eye health.

When shopping for this fruit, which has a somewhat tart flavor with over-tones of berries, choose those with unbroken and unbruised skin. A ripe kiwi yields to gentle pressure. Most kiwis are sold hard and must be ripened at home. Ripen them at room temperature, out of the sun. Refrigerate ripe kiwis for up to one week. To enjoy, peel the skin with a sharp knife or a vegetable peeler. Slice crosswise. Kiwis will not discolor when exposed to the air and are a perfect choice for salads or garnish. Heating is not recommended, however, as the kiwi turns an unappetizing shade of olive green.

I often add this luscious fruit to my morning smoothie for its rich array of vitamins, minerals, and phytonutrients, in addition to its distinctive flavor. In my kitchen, it's also a frequent companion to other fruit when I prepare a fresh fruit salad.

*See **Kiwi Melon Smoothie** recipe on page 116.*

Lemons

Although acid to the taste, the juice of a lemon is a great alkalizer for the body. When our bodies are too acid, our immune systems are compromised and our energy abates. Of all the citrus fruits, lemon is the most potent detoxifier. According to Steve Meyerowitz in his book *Power Juices Super Drinks,* lemon kills some types of intestinal parasites, such as roundworms, and dissolves gallstones.

Limonene, the volatile oil responsible for the distinctive lemon aroma and an oil that can irritate the skin in susceptible persons, even helps treat some forms of cancer such as breast cancer. If taken in the morning on an empty stomach diluted with water, lemon juice is known to improve liver function and has been used to help eliminate kidney stones. The organic acids in all citrus fruits stimulate digestive juices and relieve constipation. Added to water or fresh juice, it helps relieve colds, coughs, and sore throats. If you have dry mouth, licking a lemon or sipping unsweetened, diluted lemon juice can stimulate saliva flow. Too much lemon juice, however, if left on the teeth, can erode tooth enamel, so rinse out your mouth with pure water or brush your teeth after consuming lemon juice. Of all the citrus fruits, lemons are the highest in both vitamin C (the juice of a medium lemon has more than 30 mg) and citric acid. They also offer potassium, magnesium, calcium, and pectin.

When a recipe calls for fresh lemon zest, which is the grated outer peel, make sure it's from an organic lemon or else it might have been waxed or sprayed with chemicals. I go through 2–3 lemons per day. (Meyer lemons are my favorites.) Each morning upon awakening, I drink the juice of ½ lemon stirred into a large glass of hot water; I add ½ lemon when making fresh vegetable juices; I add lemon juice to salad dressings; and I sprinkle it on grains and vegetables. Fresh lemon juice improves the flavor of many vegetables, especially those that contain sulfur compounds, such as broccoli. Concerned about weight? Lemon juice is a perfect nonfat alternative to butter, oil dressings, and rich sauces. Invest in a good citrus juicer; it's inexpensive, user-friendly, and very practical.

*See **Fresh & Luscious Lemon Dressing** recipe on page 122.*

Medicinal, Culinary Herbs & Spices

Many people think of herbs and other spices as medicine since herbal medicine was a precursor of modern pharmacology, and about one-fourth of all prescription medicines are derived from them. The herbs and spices listed below are not as potent as some of their more medicinal cousins, but they confer some venerable health benefits—providing a wide variety of active phytochemicals that promote health and protect against chronic diseases.

- *Basil:* A favorite in ethnic dishes from Indonesia to Italy, basil has a great affinity for tomato sauce, and is savored as a pesto ingredient.

- *Chives:* A relative to the onion, this common—and rewarding—kitchen window box herb can add delicious flavors to many dishes.

- *Cilantro:* Also known as coriander, the pungent fresh leaves or seeds of this herb are basic in cuisine worldwide.

- *Dill:* An aromatic herb with delicate, lacy leaves similar in appearance to its relative, fennel, dill is widely used in pickles and salad dressings.

- *Mint:* Refreshingly cool, peppermint and spearmint are the best known of more than 2,000 varieties. Chewing the leaves can freshen breath. Spearmint is used primarily for flavoring foods.

- *Oregano:* This aromatic herb is well known to those who enjoy the delicious fragrance and taste of Italian cuisine.

- *Rosemary:* A potent member of the mint family, rosemary is available fresh and dried; and is often added to breads, dressings, and dips.

- *Sage:* The bold, almost camphorous aroma of sage becomes even more potent when dried (a small amount of dried sage goes a long way); and goes well with assertive flavors such as rosemary, thyme, and bay.

- *Thyme:* Brewed as a tea, thyme is thought to be a natural tranquilizer.

- *Turmeric:* An Indian spice, turmeric gets its yellow color from curcumin, which is said to have many healing properties, especially as an anti-inflammatory.

Mushrooms

Alongtime staple of many Asian diets, mushrooms are fat-free, very low in calories, and rich in minerals; and some varieties (such as shiitake) are rich in plant chemicals that may boost immune function. Japanese studies have shown that shiitake mushrooms help fight cancer, infections, and such auto-immune diseases as rheumatoid arthritis and lupus. They contain the phyto-nutrient lenitan, which is a biological response modifier that boosts the function of tumor-fighting interleukin-1 and cancer-cell killers known as T lymphocytes. Many leading integrative cancer therapists prescribe shiitake mushrooms to prevent the development of cancer and stop it from spreading. Some Japanese studies show that these mushrooms also may lower cholesterol and blood pressure. They are often recommended for overall rejuvenation and as an anti-aging food. I dice shiitakes and put them in soups, salads, and grain dishes. I also incorporate them into my veggie burgers.

White mushrooms and Portobellos are good sources of selenium. The mineral selenium may help prevent prostate cancer, as it is thought to work with vitamin E to clean up the free radicals that damage cells. At the City of Hope Cancer Center in Los Angeles, researchers' early laboratory findings in animals suggest that substances in the common white mushroom slow an enzyme used in the production of estrogen, which may promote cancer in postmenopausal women. I always have dried mushrooms on hand that I can hydrate quickly when I may not have time to visit a farmers' market or natural food store.

See **Mellow Mushroom Gravy** *recipe on page 126.*

Oats

Cultivated oats are native to northern Central Asia but have found a permanent home in the British Isles as well as other cold, damp climates. The U.S. domestic supply of oats is grown primarily in the northern Midwest.

The humble oat came to the forefront of the nutrition world in 1997 when the FDA allowed a label to be placed on oat foods claiming an association between consumption of a diet high in oatmeal, oat bran, or oat flour and a reduced risk for coronary heart disease—our nation's number-one killer. The overall conclusion from the FDA review was that oats could lower serum cholesterol levels, especially LDLs. According to Steven Pratt, MD, in his book *SuperFoods Rx*, the main active ingredient that yielded this exciting positive effect is the soluble fiber found in oats called "beta glucan". Oat bran became touted as the magic bullet against cholesterol, although subsequent research showed that the cholesterol-lowering effect of oat bran was less dramatic than originally thought, and the oat-bran story faded away. In any case, it's usually better and more nutritious to choose the whole food.

Pratt dignifies oats as a flagship NATUREFOOD for practical reasons: they're inexpensive, readily available, and incredibly easy to incorporate into your life. Just about all restaurants have oatmeal on their breakfast menus. They are an excellent source of complex carbohydrates (the healthy kind) that your body requires to sustain energy. They have twice as much protein as brown rice and have an amino acid content similar to that of wheat. Only the outer husk is removed during milling, so oat products retain more of their original nutrients than refined wheat products. They're also a rich source of thiamine, iron, and selenium, and contain phytonutrients that show promise as an aid to reducing heart disease and some forms of cancer.

Oats are the one adaptogen grain, meaning that they improve resistance to stress and thus support the system being in a healthy state of balance. Oats help regulate the thyroid, soothe the nervous and digestive systems, reduce the craving for cigarettes, and stabilize blood sugar. In fact, the same soluble fiber that reduces cholesterol—beta-glucan—also seems to benefit those who suffer from type II diabetes. People who eat oatmeal- or oat bran–rich foods experience lower spikes in their blood-sugar levels than they could get with foods such as white rice or white bread. The soluble fibers slow the rate at which food leaves the stomach and delays the absorption of glucose following a meal. As stabilizing blood sugar is the goal of anyone with diabetes, this is an extremely beneficial effect. One study in the *Journal of the American Medical Association* found a low intake of cereal fiber to be inversely associated with a risk for diabetes.

Oats are available in three basic forms: 1) *Whole oat groats* (about the size of long-grain rice) take as long to cook as brown rice. They're rarely cooked whole. 2) *Steel-cut oats,* my favorite ones, require less cooking time than whole oats and have a nutty, pleasing texture. Also called Scottish or Irish oats, the oat groat is cut into two or three pieces, which is how it gets its name. 3) *Rolled oats,* the most popular, are made by pressing whole oats between two rollers. They vary from old-fashioned "thick" flakes (each of which is one flattened oat groat) to tiny particles for "instant" cooking.

Oat flour yields a sweet, cake-like crumb that retains its freshness far longer than wheat-flour products because oats contain a natural antioxidant. For a dairy-free but milk-like base, use oat flour in soup, sauces, cereals, and breads. (Rolled oats, rather than oat flour, best enhance yeast breads.) I always make my own fresh oat flour from whole oats using The Kitchen Mill. In seconds, you can grind any whole grain into flour at a low temperature so that you retain all of the enzymes and nutritional value. (Refer to the section on "Setting Up Your Healthy Kitchen" on page 133.)

Onions

Whether green, red, white, yellow, or sweet, onions are members of the allium plant family, which also includes garlic, leeks, and shallots. Worldwide, the onion ranks number six as a vegetable crop; in the United States, it's number four. These versatile vegetables come in many sizes, colors, and flavors; and they are fat-, sodium-, and cholesterol-free and very low in calories. They add a taste sensation to any dish.

I admire onions for more than their flavor; their nutritional value is impressive too. The green tops of spring onions are a good source of vitamin C and beta-carotene. Onions also contain quercetin, a potent antioxidant, and sulfur compounds that lower cholesterol. Recent studies give credence to the centuries-old beliefs about onions being a heart tonic. We now know that adenosine, a substance in onions, hinders clot formation, which may help prevent heart attacks. According to the book by Reader's Digest, *Foods That Harm, Foods That Heal,* onions may protect against the artery-clogging damage of cholesterol by raising the levels of protective high-density lipoproteins (HDLs). Still other studies suggest that eating ample amounts of onions may help prevent high blood pressure.

Two of the drawbacks of eating lots of onions are the effects they have on the odor of your breath and your skin. The odor is caused by the sulfur compounds found in the onions. Perhaps you can overlook (or "oversmell") this drawback when you learn that onions also contain substances that have a mild antibacterial effect, which validates the old folk remedy of rubbing a raw onion on a cut to prevent infection.

Do you love onions but don't like what happens to your eyes when you chop or dice them? The onions' sulfur compounds combine with enzymes to form a type of sulfuric acid, which is what brings tears to the eyes. On the bright side, this effect may help clear congested nasal passages during a cold. To cut down on the tears, try putting the onion in the freezer for 15–20 minutes before cutting it, in addition to keeping your mouth open (breathe through your mouth, not your nose) while cutting.

See **Corny Onion Salad** *recipe on page 120.*

Oranges

L ong considered a favorite breakfast food, fresh orange juice, or the whole orange, is a potent source of vitamin C. The recommended daily allowance for Americans is 90 mg per day for adult males and 75 mg for adult females. This level, says Pratt (*SuperFoods Rx*), is quite low, and he recommends that the optimal intake of dietary vitamin C is 350 mg or more from food. According to his research, up to a third of us consume less than 60 mg of vitamin C daily. Among other functions, vitamin C is essential for the formation of collagen— the connective tissue matrix within our bones. A single navel orange, at only 64 calories, provides 83 mg of vitamin C, folate (plant source of folic acid), thiamine, and potassium; plus citrus flavonoids that are found in the fruit's tissue, juice, pulp, and skin. One of the flavonoids, hesperidin, is a superb antioxidant and antimutagenic. The latter refers to its ability to prevent cells from mutating and initiating one of the first steps in the development of cancer and other chronic diseases. Hesperidin also works to revive vitamin C after it has quenched a free radical. In other words, the hesperidin strengthens and amplifies the effect of vitamin C in your body. In one clinical trial, orange juice was shown to elevate HDL cholesterol ("good") while lowering LDL ("bad") cholesterol.

The sunny orange also provides beta-cryptoxanthin, a carotenoid that may help prevent colon cancer. Nobiletin, a flavonoid found in the flesh of oranges, may have anti-inflammatory actions. You're probably familiar with the pectin in oranges, the dietary fiber that's so effective that it helps to reduce cholesterol. It is present in large amounts in the white lining of citrus fruit. An easy way to increase your pectin intake is to eat the white pith. I always eat the "white stuff" on the inside of orange or tangerine rinds, scooping up a little of the orange color as well to boost my limonene intake. Limonene is an oil that may help treat some forms of cancer such as breast cancer. Oranges are a delicious snack and a flavorful ingredient in salads. Canned oranges lose most of their vitamin C and some minerals during processing and are usually packed in high-sugar syrups. Go for fresh! You can make fresh juice in seconds with a citrus juicer, although I prefer to put the entire organic orange through my more powerful juicer to garner the most nutrients.

*See **Orangey Apple Zinger Juice** recipe on page 111.*
*See **Orange Balsamic Vinaigrette** recipe on page 123.*

Parsley

T his culinary herb is so much more than a colorful garnish. It's a bona fide storehouse of synergistic nutrients that rejuvenate and detoxify the body. A good source of vitamin C, iron, calcium, sodium, beta-carotene, vanadium, manganese, and chlorophyll, parsley can be used in so many ways. Include it when you make fresh juices. One of my favorite combinations is parsley, carrots, beet, spinach, lemon, and ginger. It's very energizing and healing. Parsley juice alleviates flatulence and sweetens breath. Nibble on a few leaves when you want your breath to be sweeter. Chop it and add to grains, salads, soups, sandwiches, and whole-grain pasta dishes.

Parsley is our best source of the volatile oil apiol, which improves appetite and digestion by increasing blood circulation to the digestive tract, thereby enhancing absorption of nutrients. This luscious green herb is well known as an effective diuretic, helping to keep a healthy flow of urine and preventing kidney stones and various urinary tract ailments. Parsley contains nutritional precursors for the manufacture of adrenal hormones, so it's a great stress-buster. Other studies show parsley to be effective in slowing the aging process, reducing depression, lowering cholesterol, strengthening the kidneys, and detoxifying the cells. Many herbalists recommend parsley to relieve the symptoms of goiter and rheumatism, and to facilitate menstruation. Some say it even promotes the growth of hair, although this is not proven. I grow Italian (flat-leaf), curly-leaf parsley, and cilantro (Mexican and Chinese parsley), so I always have it fresh to use any time.

See **Rejuvenating Parsley Pear Blend** *recipe on page 114.*

Parsnips

This vegetable is from the same family as carrots and, surprisingly, is just as sweet. In fact, they even look like white/yellow carrots and have a sweet, nutty flavor that goes well with other vegetables in soups or stews. Low in calories, they also can be served as a side dish or instead of potatoes or other starchy foods. I often read that they are too fibrous to eat raw; don't believe it! They can be juiced or grated and added to salads. In fact, I make a salad of grated parsnips and carrots and add a couple of ounces of goji berries—all tossed with some fresh dressing.

Like cucumbers, watermelon, red bell peppers, and goji berries, parsnips could be nicknamed "the beauty food". The nutritional components help strengthen hair and nails and improve skin quality. Those who suffer from acne or other skin disorders will appreciate their unique balance of potassium, phosphorus, sulfur, silicon, chlorine, and vitamin C for their skin-flattering benefits. A half-cup serving has only 60 calories and is high in fiber; it also provides 300 mg of potassium and between 10% and 20% of the daily requirements of vitamin C and folate. Their chlorine and phosphorus levels improve function in the lungs and the bronchial tubes. Parsnips have been used as a diuretic, an anti-arthritic agent, and for detoxifying. I also recommend parsnip juice to help dissolve gall and kidney stones.

Often the parsnips available in supermarkets are too old and flabby and rarely worth purchasing. No wonder so few people use them today. A parsnip that is allowed to remain in the ground at least two weeks past the first frost is unbelievably sweet and satisfying, so they're best in the late fall and winter. Select ones about the size of a medium carrot; reject any that are covered with roots or are soft and shrunken. Most parsnips are sold with the tops removed; if the tops are still attached, cut them off before storing them so they don't draw moisture from the roots. Look for straight, smooth-skinned roots that are a tan or creamy-white color, firm and fresh-looking, without gray, dark, or soft spots. They can be kept for a few weeks in the refrigerator. So, the next time you buy carrots or other vegetables for juicing, mix it up. Add ½ lb. of parsnips and enjoy their sweet nutrition.

See **Skin-Beautifying Cocktail** recipe on page 112.

Pears

Once called the "butter fruit," pears come in hundreds of varieties and are scattered around the globe. Each falls into one of two categories: winter pears or Asian pears. The difference lies mainly in texture. Winter pears (a misnomer because most ripen in the fall) become succulent and juicy when ripe, while Asian pears turn crisp and crunchy like apples. In America, these seven winter pears dominate the market: Anjou, Bartlett, Red Bartlett, Bosc, Comice, Forelle, and Seckel. The trick lies in choosing the right pear for your purpose and using it at perfect ripeness, as described in an article featured in the fall 2004 issue of the magazine *Eating Well.*

- *Anjou:* The most abundant of all fresh pears, Anjous ripen without changing their light green or yellow-green color. They are ready for eating when they yield to gentle thumb pressure near the stem. The spicy taste and smooth white flesh of the Anjou is best enjoyed fresh, adding texture and interest to a salad. Season: October–June.

- *Bartlett:* Known as the "summer" pear, the Bartlett is bright yellow when ripe and sometimes sports a crimson blush. The flesh is smooth and juicy, excellent for canning, poaching, or fresh eating. Season: August–January.

- *Red Bartlett:* Similar in flavor and texture to the regular Bartlett, this variety turns a stunning red when ripe, making it perfect for fruit-bowl displays. Season: August–January.

- *Bosc:* Distinguished by its long tapering neck and slim stem, the Bosc stays golden brown into maturity. It is ready to eat when flesh near the stem feels soft. While not typically eaten out of hand, its dense flesh and buttery texture make the Bosc a great choice for poaching, roasting, broiling, or grilling. Season: August–May.

- *Comice:* Less elegant than its cousins, the Comice is stubby with a short neck. It turns from green to green-yellow when ripe, yielding to pressure. Entering its prime during the December holidays, the Comice's smooth and aromatic flesh is ideal on a nut- or seed-cheese platter. Season: August–February.

- *Forelle:* This smaller, bell-shaped variety turns golden yellow with blush spots as it ripens. Its characteristic sweet, juicy flesh makes it wonderful for fresh eating. Season: September–February.

- *Seckel:* The smallest of all pear varieties, Seckels are one-quarter the size of Bartletts—it takes several to make a snack. This tiny pear is reddish yellow or completely red when ripe. Seckels are sweet, crisp, and delicious, and they are best enjoyed eaten fresh. Season: August–February.

Pears are harvested before they are fully ripe. They will ripen as they sit at room temperature, but to speed the process, place pears in a sealed plastic bag with one or more bananas. Refrigerate ripe pears.

Now that you know how to select your pears, you should know how salubrious they are for your health. Pears contain lignin, an insoluble fiber that helps usher cholesterol out of the body. Lignin acts like Velcro, trapping cholesterol molecules in the intestine before they get absorbed into the bloodstream. And because lignin can't pass through the intestinal wall, it goes into the stool, taking cholesterol along with it, explains Mary Ellen Camire, PhD, associate professor and chair of the Department of Food Science and Human Nutrition at the

University of Maine in Orono. "Because of the lignin, eating pears on a regular basis can have a big impact on lowering cholesterol," she says.

The insoluble fiber in pears serves another useful purpose. Insoluble fiber, as the name suggests, doesn't dissolve in the intestine. What it does, however, is absorb large amounts of water. This causes stools to pass more easily and quickly through the digestive tract, which helps prevent constipation and hemorrhoids and also reduces the risk of colon cancer.

Pears contain another type of fiber, called pectin, which is the same stuff you add to jellies and jams to help them jell. Pectin is a soluble fiber, meaning that it dissolves in the intestine, forming a sticky, gel-like coating. As with lignin, pectin binds to cholesterol, causing it to be removed in the stool. When you add up all the fiber in a single, medium-sized pear, you get about 5 grams. That's quite impressive!

Pears are low in calories (about 100 calories per pear), and they boast useful amounts of vitamin C, folate, and potassium. In addition, they are low in sodium and have small amounts of phosphorus and vitamin A. Dried pears provide a more concentrated form of calories and nutrients than fresh pears. I enjoy pears all year round; when they are beautifully ripe, I quarter them and put them in plastic freezer bags, so any time of the year I can pop them into my smoothies for a delicious, nutritious pear drink. However, never store a fresh pear sealed in plastic. Without freely circulating oxygen, the core will turn brown, and brown spots will develop under the skin.

See **Pear Cashew Cream Topping** recipe on page 128.

Persimmons

The persimmon is a glossy, bright red-orange fruit that looks like a plastic tomato. When fully ripe, it delivers a pleasure sensation unlike most other fruits. Of course, an unripe persimmon is astringent, and biting into one causes one big pucker. Native to both North America and Asia, when the persimmon is mature, its flavor is a blend of plums, pumpkin, apricots, and honey. Although these beautiful gems are mainly available in the late fall and early winter, I manage to enjoy them year round.

Eat a persimmon as you would eat a ripe papaya—out of hand. Cut the persimmon in half and spoon out the heavenly soft flesh, add it to a fruit salad or smoothie, or purée it for dips and fresh-fruit sauces. For another delectable treat, halve a fully ripe persimmon, wrap it tightly in plastic, and freeze it for at least four hours and you have a no-fuss, healthful persimmon "sherbet". Simply eat it out of the shell with a spoon. I also take ripe persimmons, cut them in ¼-inch slices, and dry them in my food dehydrator. When the fruit is fully dried, I usually put them in freezer plastic bags and keep them in the freezer to enjoy all year long, either dried or rehydrated in water. Unlike most other dried fruits, persimmons hold their brilliant gold color without the assistance of sulfur treatment. And, of course, there's always persimmon pudding—a favorite during the holidays.

The Asian persimmon originated in China. It is widely cultivated by the Japanese, who consider it their national fruit. The large *Tanenashi* and the *Hachiya* are pointed like an acorn at their base. Both become very soft when ripe. The smaller, tomato-shaped *Fuyu* is nonastringent and remains firm when ripe. Select plump fruits that have a smooth skin, intact green cap, and are soft (Fuyu excepted).

Persimmons are a good source of vitamin A and potassium, containing 60% more potassium than orange juice. In fact, one persimmon, with only 118 calories, provides 3,640 IU of vitamin A, 270 mg of potassium, and 6g of fiber.

*See **Perfectly Persimmon Smoothie** recipe on page 115.*

Pomegranates

This dark red fruit is "hot" these days, especially in the form of pomegranate juice. Pomegranates abound with disease-fighting antioxidants; some studies show that they offer almost three times the antioxidants of such well-known antioxidant super sources as green tea, red wine, blueberry juice, cranberry juice, and orange juice. Additionally, pomegranates contain potassium, fiber, vitamin C, and niacin, all of which can contribute to increased energy and good health. It also can boast some more specific heart-healthy benefits. Research reported in the *American Journal of Clinical Nutrition* (2000, 71:1062) showed that pomegranate juice reduced plaque build-up in arteries by 44% when given to subjects.

Here is what some scientific journals are saying about pomegranate juice: ". . . pomegranate juice consumption can offer a wide protection against cardiovascular disease" *(Atherosclerosis)*; ". . . pomegranate juice can contribute to the reduction of oxidative stress and atherogenesis" (*The Journal of Nutrition*); and "Pomegranate juice treatment significantly and substantially inhibited the progression of atherosclerotic lesions [in mice]" (*The American Journal of Clinical Nutrition*).

Pomegranate juice is one of my all-time favorite beverages. I used to juice this fruit until I found the perfect source at my local farmers' market. So now, once each week, I purchase two gallons of the freshly squeezed, raw juice. (You often can find pasteurized pomegranate juice at health-food stores, both bottled by itself, and as an ingredient in blended fruit beverages.) In addition to drinking this colorful elixir, I also make lots of frozen cubes from the juice to put in my water, in smoothies, and in soups as part of the liquid base for chilled fruit soups. I also enjoy sucking on the frozen pomegranate cubes as a wonderful snack or dessert treat. Besides the normal-shaped ice-cube trays, I also have some in the shapes of hearts, stars, fruit, flowers, teddy bears, and other animals. A heart of frozen pomegranate juice, or other fruit juice, is a lovely, special touch in a glass of water, tea, or juice.

The pulp (seed) of the pomegranate fruit is 82% water and contains 63 calories per 100 grams of the edible portion. One pomegranate provides most of the body's daily potassium and vitamin-C needs, a healthy dose of fiber, and no fat. Next to pure water, lemon water, and the water from a young coconut, fresh pomegranate juice is one of my favorite, healthful beverages that I have several times each week when it is available in season.

See **Pomegranate Fruit Smoothie** recipe on page 119.

Raspberries

Raspberries belong to the rose family. That explains why they grow on bramble bushes with prickly stems. But despite these prickles, there are few pleasures on a midsummer's afternoon that are as sweet or as healthful as eating raspberries picked fresh off the bush.

Raspberries—both wild and cultivated—are low in calories (one cup contains only 60 calories) and high in vitamin C (30 mg in a cup). This same amount also provides 30 mcg of folate, 190 mg of potassium, and some iron. The vitamin-C content increases the iron's absorption, although this may be offset by the oxalic acid in raspberries, which binds with this mineral. Raspberries have more fiber than most other fruits; the 7 grams of fiber in each cup are double the amount found in strawberries. The seeds in these little gems provide insoluble fiber that helps prevent constipation. Each raspberry is actually a small cluster of 75 to 125 fiber-rich seeds, with every seed encased in a tiny, juicy lobe of its own. The fruit is also high in pectin, a form of soluble fiber that helps control blood-cholesterol levels.

Raspberries are one of the top antioxidant foods. They contain the same cancer-fighting ellagic acid as strawberries, but they have 50% more of it. In addition, raspberries contain anthocyanins, antioxidant plant pigments that have been shown to prevent cancer and heart disease.

Raspberries spoil faster than most berries because of their delicate structure and hollow core. Once picked, they should be eaten as soon as possible. Before buying raspberries, check that all of them, not just the ones on top, are in good condition; even then, they mold quickly and should be used within 24 hours. Freezing, however, will preserve them for up to a year. Most cultivated raspberries are red, but there are also varieties in yellow, apricot, amber, and purple (or "black")—all similar in flavor and texture. When they are in season, I buy raspberries in all of these colors at local farmers' markets. Berries, when in season and organically grown, are a great food to eat as a mono-diet (just one food all day long) to cleanse and rejuvenate your body.

If you are sensitive to aspirin, you also may react to raspberries, which contain a natural salicylate that is similar to the major ingredient in aspirin. Raspberries contain oxalic acid, which can precipitate kidney and bladder stones in susceptible people; however, it would take a very large amount of raspberries to create problems.

Sea Vegetables

Ounce for ounce, sea vegetables are a valuable treatment for *Candida albicans,* as well as other immune-compromised diseases such as chronic fatigue, HIV infection, arthritis, and allergies. My three favorite sea vegetables (and the ones that I use most often in my diet, in my healthful-food cooking classes, and in my private culinary instruction) are dulse, kelp, and nori.

Nori *(Porphyra tenera)* is my favorite sea vegetable. It has the highest protein content of all the seaweeds—higher than soybeans, milk, meat, fish, or poultry—and is the most easily digested. It is very high in vitamins A (more than carrots), B (B_1 and niacin), C, and D, and the minerals calcium, iodine, iron, potassium, phosphorus, and many trace elements. It is also low in calories (only 10 per sheet), high in fiber, and contains an enzyme that helps break down cholesterol deposits. Some of the healing properties of nori include the following: may help treat painful urination, goiter, edema, high blood pressure, cough with green or yellow mucus, fatty cysts under the skin, and warts; and may aid in digestion, especially with fried foods. It's a diuretic and all-around terrific health food.

- *Nori*, called *laver* when it is cultivated, has one of the sweeter flavors of the seaweeds. You're probably familiar with the sheets of nori used to wrap and hold rice, vegetables, and raw or cooked fish in small rolls (sushi) that can be eaten with the hands. I put my salad ingredients in the nori sheets and wrap them up like a burrito. I also cut out smaller nori squares (about 4-inch squares) and put a dollop of hummus or other spreads in the center along with some julienned vegetables (such as carrots, cucumbers, bell peppers) and sprouts, and eat three or four of these for a meal or snack. Nori also can be crumbled, chopped, broken, or cut with scissors and added to soups, salads, dressings, spreads, stews, or desserts. It's even a frequent ingredient in my vegetable smoothies.

- *Dulse* (*Palmaria palmata*) is an especially rich source of potassium, iron, iodine, vitamin B_6, riboflavin, and dietary fiber; and provides a complete array of minerals, trace elements, enzymes, and phytochemicals, as well as some high-quality vegetable protein. My favorite way to incorporate dulse into my food program is in a granule form which I get at my local health-food store. Whether you buy it loose or packaged, by itself or mixed with garlic and other herbs, it's a great way to spice up your diet and detoxify at the same time. It's delicious sprinkled over spinach, popcorn, brown rice, and with walnuts. I also use it in soups, salads, dressings, dips, sauces, tabouli, potatoes, beans, and more. It is a supremely balanced nutrient with 300 times more iodine and 50 times more iron than wheat. Research indicates it may fight the herpes virus. It has purifying and tonic effects on the body, yet its natural, balanced salts nourish as a mineral, without inducing thirst.

- *Kelp* (*Laminaria*) is a stellar, nutrient-dense sea vegetable that is especially rich in potassium, iron, iodine, riboflavin, dietary fiber, and vitamins A, B, C, D, E, and K. It also contains a natural substance that enhances flavor and tenderizes, and sodium alginate (algin), an element that helps remove radioactive particles and heavy metals from the body. Algin, carrageenan, and agar are kelp gels that rejuvenate gastrointestinal health and aid digestion. Kelp works as a blood purifier, relieves the stiffness of arthritis, and promotes adrenal, pituitary, and thyroid health. Its natural iodine can normalize thyroid-related disorders such as abnormal weight gain and lymph system congestion. As a demulcent, it soothes and protects mucous membranes and even may help eliminate herpes outbreaks.

The next time you want a healthful seasoning, instead of salt, reach for kelp granules. I enjoy them plain and mixed with cayenne or garlic (available in health-food stores).

Sesame Seeds and Tahini

The minute size of sesame seeds belies their remarkable nutritional value. In Oriental medicine, sesame seeds are used to build a deficient liver and kidneys when there are symptoms of premature graying, dizziness, and general weakness. Available in cream-colored and black, sesame seeds contain over 35% protein, more than any nut or seed. They are about 50% oil and are high in vitamin D, which makes sesame oil and butter highly stable and resistant to oxidation. Sesame contains as much iron as liver, and it's a good source of phosphorus, niacin, thiamine, magnesium, zinc, and omega-3 fatty acids. It has a unique surplus of two amino acids, methionine and tryptophan, which are usually lacking in popular vegetable protein foods.

In one cup of sesame seeds, you'll find about 875 calories (obviously you won't eat a cup of seeds), 17 grams of fiber, 1,400 mg of calcium, 880 mg of phosphorus, 600 mg of potassium, and 100 IU of vitamin A. They also contain lignans—an antioxidant. Sesame seeds are available hulled or unhulled. Hulled sesame seeds lose their fiber and much of their potassium, iron, and vitamins A and B6, folate, and thiamine. If the hulls are removed with caustic alkali rather than mechanically, the nutrient loss is even greater.

While sesame seeds are an excellent source of calcium, this calcium is bonded with oxalic acid, and not easily bioavailable. Soaking the seeds overnight and then toasting them reduces their oxalic acid content. While hulling the seeds actually eliminates the oxalic acid, it also eliminates most of the calcium. Personally, I eat unhulled seeds raw, unsoaked and soaked, and am not concerned with calcium loss with all of the other calcium-rich foods I consume. Whole sesame seeds enjoyed in moderation should not interfere with calcium absorption in healthy individuals.

If purchasing hulled sesame seeds, purchase only those that have had their hulls mechanically removed. If the hulled seeds are not organic, you can assume that caustic lye was used to de-hull them, thus denaturing nutrients and flavor. I use whole sesame seeds (black and cream-colored) in salads, vegetable dishes, and condiments, and in baking. Washing the seeds removes any bitter taste, and toasting them enhances their flavor. To wash, place the seeds in a bowl and fill with water; pour the seeds into a strainer, being careful to not pour out any of the sand or grit (if there is any) that may have settled in the bottom of the bowl. After soaking, I dry my seeds in a dehydrator at a low temperature, so I save the enzymes and nutrients.

The black sesame seed is more richly flavored and a feast for the eyes when used whole or ground in dishes or as a seed-butter. The stronger flavor of black sesame seeds indicates that they are higher in minerals and trace nutrients than the lighter-colored sesame seeds. I encourage you, however, to purchase only organic black sesame seeds or butter. The "black" sesame seeds sometimes found in Asian markets are dyed a shiny, monochromatic black. Unadulterated ones have a dull, matte finish and range in color from coal black to gray-black, with an occasional rust-colored seed.

Tahini is a creamy-smooth paste ground from hulled raw or roasted sesame seeds (as opposed to pure sesame butter, which is ground from whole, or unhulled, sesame seeds). This high-protein spread is a culinary staple in Middle Eastern and some Asian cultures and is a popular ingredient used in dressings, sauces, and desserts. Tahini is a common ingredient in halvah, hummus (although it can be made without tahini), and baba ghanoush. I use it as a base in salad dressings along with some water, lime or lemon juice, pressed garlic, minced fresh herbs such as oregano, cilantro, or parsley, and Celtic sea salt (optional). Because sesame butter and tahini are high in vitamin E, they have a longer shelf life than other nut and seed butters. Once opened, sesame butter/tahini should be refrigerated, where it will hold for about six months. If it tastes or smells harsh, it is rancid and should be discarded. Try both light-colored and black sesame butters available in health-food stores.

See **Sesame Milk** *recipe on page 110.*
See **Grapefruit Tahini Dressing** *recipe on page 122.*
See **Tahini Salsa Dressing** *recipe on page 124.*

Spinach

Popeye wasn't just a muscular cartoon figure; he knew what he was talking about when it came to this strength- and energy-building miracle food. This green goddess food is really one of the best body builders, cleansers, and rejuvenators you can eat. One of my favorite leafy green vegetables (along with romaine lettuce, arugala, and sunflower sprout greens), spinach is among the best sources of folate, which is critically important for cardiovascular and brain health. Low folic-acid levels in your blood are associated with high levels of the amino acid homocysteine. Excessive homocysteine is a marker for increased risk of death resulting from heart disease. And since heart disease is a strong risk factor for memory loss, high levels of homocysteine are a marker for Alzheimer's disease as well. A half cup of boiled spinach contains 130 mcg of folate out of the 400 mcg you need to eat every day to keep your homocysteine levels under control. In a recent report, neurologists recommended eating spinach three times per week as a brain tonic.

Spinach also contains nearly twice as much iron as most other greens. Iron enables our red blood cells to carry more oxygen, which strengthens all cells—especially those of the brain and the respiratory system. Because of its high iron content, spinach is a valuable food for the treatment of anemia, circulatory weaknesses, and cholesterol diseases such as hypertension and stroke.

Do you want an excellent food to support eye health? You can't go wrong with spinach. It contains an abundance of the two carotenoids mentioned previously, zeaxanthin and lutein, which help prevent age-related macular degeneration and retard the development of cataracts. As with other green vegetables high in carotene, spinach plays a significant role against cancer. In one epidemiological study, women who consumed spinach regularly had a lower incidence of cervical cancer. Pratt selected spinach as one of the 14 healthiest foods you can eat. It is one of the only two vegetables with a significant amount of coenzyme Q_{10}; the other is broccoli. Coenzyme Q_{10} works in synergy with vitamins C, E, and glutathione. (Glutathione is the main antioxidant in cells. It is found in the watery interior of cells, where it protects DNA from oxidation.) Coenzyme Q_{10} is a key player in our skin's antioxidant defense mechanism against sunlight damage and also a significant player in mitochondrial energy production. (The mitochondria are the cells' energy factories.) Spinach is an important source of this critical antioxidant.

The minerals found in spinach are highly alkaline, which helps our bodies fight uric acid build-up and the symptoms of aging that go along with it. But spinach is also high in oxalic acid, which interferes with calcium absorption. (We are better able to metabolize this acid when we eat the spinach uncooked.)

Every week, I buy a three-pound box of organic, baby-leaf spinach at my local farmers' market. I blend it for dips, soups, and vegetable smoothies, juice it with other vegetables, and eat it daily in salads. With all due respect to Popeye, eat fresh spinach, not canned! Put a nice big handful of fresh, crisp, dark spinach leaves into your salad bowl or into your juicer or blender. This chlorophyll-rich

NATUREFOOD is best when grown organically because conventionally grown spinach is one of the ten most pesticide-laden vegetables.

Strawberries

Heart-shaped and red, this tiny jewel, the strawberry, has long been thought of as a symbol of love. In the language of symbolism, it represents perfection and righteousness. According to James Joseph, PhD, in his book *The Color Code,* throughout history, strawberries were served at important state occasions to promote peace and prosperity. In France, strawberries were traditionally regarded as an aphrodisiac. So great was the belief in their powers that newlyweds were served delicate red strawberry soup. And if a man and woman split a double strawberry, custom held that they would fall in love. Until recently, scientists might have dismissed all this lore as hocus-pocus. But now we know that there really is reason to extol the virtues of the healing power of strawberries.

Low in calories—about 40 per cup—strawberries are very high in vitamin C. In fact, weight for weight, they are a better source of this vitamin than oranges. One cup contains about 90 mg, or 100% of the RDA for adults. They are also a good source of folate (30 mcg in one cup), with 3 grams of fiber, 250 mg of potassium, and fair amounts of silicon, B-complex, and iron. Furthermore, they are a good source of pectin and other soluble fibers that help lower cholesterol. Even the seeds in strawberries provide insoluble fiber, which helps prevent constipation; however, they can be irritating to people with such intestinal disorders as inflammatory bowel disease or diverticulosis, a condition in which small pouches bulge outward along the intestinal wall.

Strawberries are a rich source of bioflavonoids, including red anthocyanin and phenolic acids. One of the phenolic acids, *ellagic acid,* may actually change a person's genetic predisposition to cancer. An analysis of recent medical-school research shows that ellagic acid kills cervical cancer cells in particular and performs similarly on cancer cells in the breast, pancreas, esophagus, skin, colon, and prostate. Many more studies have shown the anticancer effect of ellagic acid and its protective effect against radiation damage to chromosomes.

Strawberries also have a tranquilizing effect; that's why surgical gloves for dentists and masks for children's anesthesia are often perfumed with a strawberry scent. A kitchen remedy to remove tartar and strengthen teeth is to rub a halved strawberry on the teeth and gums and leave it on for 45 minutes. Rinse with warm water. They also are said to whiten teeth and are used to get rid of garlic breath. And if that weren't enough, the Chinese claim that a handful of the red berries is a cure for a hangover.

Whatever reasons you choose to enjoy these red gems, pick out strawberries with fresh green stems attached and a bright red color throughout. Pale or yellowish berries are unripe and sour. Because they contain the aspirin-like compound salicylate, as well as a common allergen, some people are allergic to strawberries. It's best to purchase organic varieties because commercially grown strawberries may contain relatively high levels of pesticide residues. I eat them as a snack (or mono-meal) by themselves and also use them in smoothies (fresh or frozen), soups, dips, and sauces.

See **Strawberry Banana Smoothie** *recipe on page 118.*

Sunflower Seeds

One of my early mentors and friends in holistic medicine was the late Paavo Airola, PhD, author of many best-selling health books. Dr. Airola suggested that one of the staples of the human diet should be seeds and nuts, but because of their high fat content, he always emphasized that we shouldn't overeat these foods. A little bit goes a long way when it comes to seeds and nuts. According to Dr. Airola's research, all seeds and nuts should be eaten raw. One of his favorite seeds was the sunflower. They can be sprinkled on salads, made into sunflower-seed butter or seed milk, made into delicious sprouts, or ground into a meal. Like most seeds and nuts, sunflower seeds are rich in vitamin E and potassium and high in minerals, including calcium, iron, magnesium, and zinc. One ounce of sunflower seeds contains about 75% of the RDA for vitamin E. They also are rich in selenium, copper, fiber, folate, and vitamin B₆. Sunflower-seed butter makes a delicious high-protein salad dressing when blended with some lemon juice and purified water, fresh garlic, one tomato, and your favorite herbs. Moreover, it's a great replacement for peanut butter on sandwiches and packed into the groove of celery. Make friends with these health-promoting seeds.

If you don't grow sunflower-sprout greens from unhulled seeds, look for them in the health-food store. They are one of the best NATUREFOODS you can eat. I put them in smoothies, mix them in salads, and snack on them just as they are—delicious and nutritious. They usually can be found in the cooled vegetable section next to the other fresh sprouts.

See **Sunflower Seed Milk** recipe on page 110.

Sweet Potatoes

Although sweet potatoes are sometimes mistakenly called yams, they are not related. True yams are an entirely different kind of tuber. However, in the southern United States, a sweet potato is called a yam. To further the confusion, canned sweet potatoes are often called yams. Also, although they are called potatoes, they are not in the same family as the common white potato. Whatever you choose to call them, these richly colored, heavenly potatoes are naturally sweet and highly nutritious. Like other brightly colored orange-yellow vegetables, they also are an excellent source of beta-carotene, a powerful antioxidant linked to lowered risk of heart disease and certain cancers. On average, one medium sweet potato provides more than 100% of the RDA for vitamin A, about ⅓ of the RDA for vitamin C and B₆, and 540 mg of potassium, along with folate (plant source of folic acid) and some iron. Sweet potatoes also contain plant sterols, compounds that can help lower cholesterol. When eaten with its skin, a sweet potato is an excellent source of soluble and insoluble fiber, which helps reduce cholesterol and may prevent diverticulosis.

Salutary sweet potatoes can boost your vitality year-round. Try them juiced (I combine their juice with a blend of vegetable juices for a "Carotenoid Cocktail", see page 113), steamed, baked, puréed, and mashed with a combination of yams and russet potatoes. I also enjoy the cooked flesh in smoothies.

See **Chocolate Sweet Potato Smoothie** *recipe on page 116.*
See **Spicy Sweet Potato Bisque** *recipe on page 130.*

Tea

To some, tea is more than just a beverage; it's a vaccine. As far back as the sixth century, tea was considered a remedy for headaches, kidney trouble, poor digestion, and ulcers. In the past decade, sales of tea in the United States have doubled as Americans seeking healthier lifestyles have turned to the beverage for its health benefits. Black and green teas come from the same plant, but they are processed differently and contain different antioxidants. Consider drinking both (perhaps alternating days) to get the greatest disease protection. Here's how Pratt describes tea. How about a NatureFood that's cheap, has no calories, is associated with relaxation and pleasure, tastes good, and is available everywhere, from the finest restaurants to the local diner? How about a food that lowers blood pressure, helps prevent cancer and osteoporosis, lowers your risk for stroke, plays a role in preventing sunlight damage to the skin (such as wrinkles and skin cancer), and contributes to your daily fluid needs? And what if, to boot, it were anti-viral, anti-inflammatory, anti-cavity, anti-allergy, and prevented cataracts? Wow! This is why I often use and recommend green, black, or white tea instead of water or juice as your liquid in smoothies and other drinks.

Tea contains more than 4,000 chemical compounds. The ones that have drawn the most attention, and which have proven benefits, include the phytonutrient polyphenols called flavonoids—the same types that are found in berries. The most potent polyphenol in tea is a substance known as epigallocatechin gallate, or EGCG, which belongs to a group of flavonoid phytochemicals known as catechins. Research has shown that the catechins are more effective antioxidants than even the powerful vitamins C and E. Tea may also prevent your bones from weakening as you age. According to a study published in 2002 in *Archives of Internal Medicine*, people who drank 2 or more cups of tea—green, black, or white (all of which come from the same plant)—daily for six to ten years had higher bone density than those who didn't drink tea regularly.

Pratt recommends having a cup of green or black tea before you exercise in the morning. The flavonoids begin to appear in your blood within about 30 minutes, giving you an antioxidant boost and thus preparing your body to handle the free radicals generated by exercise. Needless to say, I have adopted this great idea into my health program. I also use black and green tea leaves to soothe minor cuts, treat sunburns, refresh puffy eyes, and soak tired feet. They also can be used to help heal fever blisters, ease toothaches, and soothe bee stings. Dip a tea bag in boiling water, squeeze out the extra moisture, and let it cool to a comfortable temperature. Then apply the bag as a compress to the affected area. Keep a couple of your favorite tea bags with you so you can take advantage of a delicious drink or their healing properties anywhere, any time. If you prefer, you can get the benefits of tea sans caffeine; just look for decaffeinated brands.

Tomatoes

Like the watermelon, this beautiful, low-calorie fruit is over 90% water. It's alkaline and jam-packed with nutrients and phytochemicals. Whether in sauce, soup, or atop a salad, tomatoes are loved by most Americans. They provide vitamin C, potassium, chromium, biotin, lutein and zeaxanthin, alpha- and beta-carotene, the B vitamins (B$_6$, niacin, folate, thiamine, and pantothenic acid), and lots of lycopene. Lycopene (in addition to being a pigment that contributes to the tomato's red color) is a member of the carotenoid family and an important part of the antioxidant defense network of the skin. In combination with other nutrients, it can raise the sun-protection factor (SPF) of the skin. Pratt extols this virtue of the tomato, and recommends eating them (raw, cooked, or processed) to enhance your skin's ability to withstand the assault from the damaging rays of the sun. It acts like an internal sunblock.

Numerous epidemiological studies have found that people who eat lots of tomatoes are significantly less likely to get cancer (according to a review published in the *Journal of the National Cancer Institute* in 1999). Study results were strongest for prostate, lung, and stomach cancer, although there's some evidence that tomatoes protect against breast, ovarian, and other cancers too. Lycopene again appears to be the source of the protective benefit.

Pratt cites many studies revealing that lycopene also may benefit your heart. Cooked tomatoes, like those in sauce, contain more absorbable lycopene than raw tomatoes. Look for organically grown, vine-ripened tomatoes in your health-food store or farmer's market for the best taste other than those from home gardens. Eat them just like an apple. They make a delicious snack and thirst-quenching treat. And because most of the nutritional value is contained in the skin, ounce for ounce, cherry tomatoes afford more nutritional value than large tomatoes.

See **Sensational Salsa** *recipe on page 124.*
See **Golden Gazpacho Soup** *recipe on page 130.*

Walnuts

A versatile and delicious nut, walnuts are the flagship nut because only they provide *two* heart-healthy essential fatty acids: linolenic and linoleic fatty acids. Linolenic acid (an omega-3 fatty acid) is associated with a lower risk of coronary artery disease, according to a study published in the *American Journal of Clinical Nutrition* in 2001. Linoleic acid may reduce your chances of having a stroke, according to a study published in *Stroke* in 2002. Several clinical trials have found that eating walnuts lowers cholesterol. For example, men and women who ate about 2 oz. of walnuts daily for a month significantly lowered their total cholesterol. The plant sterols in walnuts play a significant role in lowering serum cholesterol levels.

Walnuts are a good source of fiber and protein, and they also provide magnesium, copper, folate, and vitamin E. Walnuts have the highest overall antioxidant activity of all nuts. One of the main antioxidants is polyphenol, which may help prevent heart disease. Nuts are high in calories, but they have many extraordinary health benefits and can be an important addition to your diet. Pratt recommends eating a handful of nuts about five times per week. He says that this simple act would reduce your chances of getting a heart attack by at least 15% and possibly as much as 51%. Choose nuts that are fresh and raw, not roasted and salted. Walnuts are superb alone or incorporated in trail mix and sandwiches, chopped and sprinkled on salads and vegetables, added to whole-grain cookies and breads, and blended in smoothies and soups. Check out my website for some blender recipes.

See ***Vanilla Orange Cream*** *recipe on page 127.*
See ***Omega-3 Walnut-Flax Topping*** *recipe on page 127.*

Watermelon

A classic picnic food, enjoyed out of doors, especially by children and participants of seed-spitting contests, watermelon is about 90% water and comes in red or yellow flesh, with or without seeds. It's one of the most cleansing foods you can eat—because of its high water content—and is also one of the finest diuretics in the plant kingdom. The zinc content of watermelons makes them an important kidney and bladder cleanser and, in fact, contributes to overall urogenital and prostate health. Watermelon lowers blood pressure in hypertension patients and eliminates toxins. According to Steve Meyerowitz, in his book *Power Juices Super Drinks,* when you juice the rind and seed (it's always best to select organic melons when juicing the rind and seed), you release a veritable "fountain of youth" of therapeutic plant compounds. It becomes a free-radical scavenger that re-oxygenates cells and acts effectively as an anti-aging agent.

Surprisingly, watermelon has only half the sugar (5%) of an apple. It tastes much sweeter, though, because sugar is its main taste-producing element—the rest is primarily water. This makes it a popular diet food and an unexcelled cooling food; it's even more cooling than cantaloupe. Watermelon relieves thirst and edema. It's a good source of vitamins C and A and the mineral potassium. And what will be music to your ears if you are interested in dropping a clothes size or two, watermelon also is low in sodium and calories and has no fat.

Watermelon contains some powerful antioxidants too. This delectable summer fruit is rich in beta-cryptoxanthin, a carotenoid that's associated with reduced risk of heart disease. And it's one of the few good sources of lycopene, a free-radical scavenger that may lower cancer and heart-disease risk (lycopene also is found in tomatoes). Unlike tomatoes, however, watermelons don't need to be cooked to provide the most absorbable form of lycopene. Watermelons also provide high amounts of glutathione, an anticancer, antioxidant, and anti-aging phytonutrient.

This heavy fruit ranges from from a few pounds in weight to as much as 40 pounds. It doesn't stand up to cooking or mincing, so use large chunks in combination with other fruit ingredients if making a salad. Watermelon can be made into a delectable smoothie (I add ginger too) or fruit soup. Three to four times each summer, I engage in a watermelon cleanse where I eat only watermelon for one to three days or choose different melons each day, such as watermelon, cantaloupe, and honeydew.

If purchasing a cut watermelon, avoid one with immature white seeds, pale flesh, or white streaks. If over-mature, its flesh is mealy and either dry or watery.

If purchasing whole, the rind should look dull, not shiny. The melon should feel heavy for its size. It will store at room temperature up to seven days whole and up to three days in the refrigerator, cut.

See **Watermelon Ginger Refresher** *recipe on page 114.*

* * *

V

RADIANT HEALTH
AT A GLANCE

HOW *NATUREFOODS* KEEP YOU HEALTHY

Research shows that these 50 foods improve your health in the following ways:

MA   *mollifies arthritis*
PC   *prevents cancer*
HD   *staves off heart disease*
WL   *supports weight loss*

BI   *boosts immunity*
EV   *enhances vision*
SA   *slows aging*
BS   *beautifies skin*

IA   *increases antioxidants*
BF   *improves brain function and memory*

	MA	PC	HD	WL	BI	EV	SA	BS	IA	BF
Almonds		•	•							
Apples		•	•	•						•
Asparagus			•						•	
Avocados		•	•			•	•	•		
Bananas			•					•		
Beans		•	•	•					•	
Beets		•	•						•	
Bell Peppers				•				•		
Blueberries		•		•			•		•	•
Broccoli		•	•	•	•					•
Brussels Sprouts		•		•		•		•		
Cantaloupe		•						•	•	
Carrots		•	•		•	•		•	•	
Celery	•	•		•						
Chili Peppers	•	•	•	•					•	
Cinnamon			•				•			
Coconut	•		•	•	•			•		
Cranberries			•							
Cucumbers	•		•	•				•		
Figs			•					•		
Flaxseed	•	•	•	•	•	•	•	•	•	•

	MA	PC	HD	WL	BI	EV	SA	BS	IA	BF
Garlic		•	•		•				•	•
Ginger	•	•	•						•	
Goji Berries					•		•	•	•	
Grapefruit	•	•	•						•	
Green Leafy Vegatables	•	•	•	•	•	•	•	•	•	•
Kale	•	•	•	•	•	•	•	•	•	•
Kiwi			•			•			•	
Lemons		•						•	•	
Medicinal Herbs & Spices	•	•	•	•	•	•	•	•	•	•
Mushrooms	•	•	•	•	•		•		•	
Oats			•							
Onions		•	•						•	
Oranges		•	•		•			•	•	
Parsley	•						•		•	
Parsnips	•							•		
Pears	•	•	•	•						
Persimmons						•		•	•	
Pomegranates		•	•		•				•	
Raspberries		•	•	•	•				•	
Sea Vegetables	•			•	•			•	•	
Sesame Seeds/Tahini								•	•	
Spinach	•	•	•	•	•	•	•	•	•	•
Strawberries		•	•					•	•	
Sunflower Seeds/Sprouts			•					•	•	
Sweet Potatoes			•			•		•	•	
Tea	•	•	•	•		•	•	•	•	
Tomatoes		•	•		•	•		•	•	
Walnuts			•							
Watermelon		•	•				•	•	•	

VI

RECIPES

42 NatureFood Recipes

"Choose what is best; habit will soon render it agreeable and easy."
— **Pythagorus**

This recipe section will introduce you to some of the endless recipes and variations possible with the 50 nutritionally superb NatureFoods that I have just described. Making and enjoying some of these nutritious treats each day will do wonders for your waistline and help you create the radiantly healthy and vibrantly energized life of your dreams. I have grouped the recipes into general sections—nut and seed milks, juices and blends, smoothies, salads, dips and dressings, and soups—but you soon will see how easy it is to modify them and put them into entirely different categories. Experiment often and your skill and satisfaction will grow boundlessly.

I've used a wide variety of foods and preparation styles so that you will have plenty of colorful, antioxidant-rich, plant-based recipes to jump-start your nutritional transformation. Learning to make good food choices is a big step toward better health and enjoyment of life. *Practice every day!* Soon you will be effortlessly disease-proofing your body as you naturally gravitate toward these NatureFoods. I encourage you to make a commitment for 30 days—just one month—and incorporate as many of these foods as possible into your diet. You will look better than you have in years and also will feel more youthful and empowered. Your family and friends will be amazed at the new you . . . *and so will you!*

Nut & Seed Milks

Use these delicious "milks" in any recipes that call for the use of dairy milk.

Sunflower Seed Milk

Makes about 4 cups

1 cup raw, shelled organic sunflower seeds
3 cups pure water
1–2 tbsp. sweetener (such as pitted dates, agave, stevia, maple syrup, or date sugar)

First, put the seeds in the blender and start grinding. Blend them dry (no liquid) until they become the consistency of nut meal. Now blend in the water. (If you like your milk to be light and smooth, pour the liquid through a strainer. If you prefer a thicker consistency, like that of a milk shake, skip the straining.) Sweeten to taste. You also may adjust the consistency by increasing or decreasing the amount of water. You can use this seed milk in any recipe that calls for milk.

Sesame Milk

Makes about 5 cups

2 cups sesame seeds, soaked for 8 hours (overnight)
2½ cups purified water

Rinse and drain the seeds. Blend the seeds and water on high speed for 20 seconds. Using a fine-mesh strainer or a seed-cheese bag, strain the seed milk. You can use the remaining leftover seed pulp for tahini.

VARIATION: You can make cashew nut milk the same way by replacing the sesame seeds with sunflower seeds. These seed and nut milks can replace dairy milk in your diet. They can be easily sweetened or enhanced with vanilla bean or extract. They make a great base for smoothies to replace water or juice.

Almond Milk

Makes about 5 cups

1 cup raw almonds (organic, if possible)
6 cups purified water (preferably distilled)

Soak the raw almonds in 2 cups of water for at least 6 hours (the first step in sprouting). In a blender, add the presoaked and drained almonds to 4 cups of water. Blend on high until creamy. If you prefer your almond milk more like the consistency of dairy milk, strain it through a fine strainer or cheese cloth to remove the fiber. Almond milk keeps 3-4 days in the refrigerator. Chill and serve.

VARIATION: To sweeten, add stevia, date sugar, pure maple syrup, or a few pitted dates and blend. If you add raw carob powder, you get "chocolate milk". I also like my almond milk with a sprinkle of cinnamon powder and a touch of vanilla extract or vanilla bean. You also can substitute sunflower seeds or cashews for the almonds, but you don't need to soak either of them if you don't have the time.

Juices & Blends

These powerful drinks encourage detoxification, which helps prevent disease.

Orangey Apple Zinger Juice

Serves 2

4 apples, cored (I prefer Fuji)
4 oranges, peeled
½ inch fresh ginger coin
Dash of cinnamon

Keep the white pith on the oranges. Juice the apples, oranges, and ginger. Pour into the glasses and sprinkle a dash of cinnamon on top.

Skin-Beautifying Cocktail

Serves 2 to 3

2 parsnips
3 carrots
1 cucumber
1 red bell pepper
2¼ lemons
4–8 leaves of romaine lettuce

Juice all ingredients and serve immediately.

Variation: Add spinach in place of the romaine. To give it more of a zingy taste, juice some ginger root (about ¼ inch coin) and/or sprinkle in a dash of cayenne pepper to the juice mixture. To make a delicious soup, take this juice mixture and blend it with a few tomatoes and, if you can find them, a cup of sunflower sprout greens.

Warm Apple Cider

Serves 3 to 4

10 apples
1 vanilla pod
1 cinnamon stick
5 orange slices
3 lemon slices
1 tsp. five-spice powder

Juice the apples and put the juice in a clear glass serving jug. Coarsely chop the vanilla pod, and break up the cinnamon stick. Combine all the other ingredients into the juice and allow the ingredients to mix and commingle in the sunshine for one hour. If sunshine is unavailable, warm on top of your clothes dryer or on the stove with low heat, making sure the mixture doesn't get too hot to touch.

Carotenoid Cocktail

Serves 1

3 carrots
1 tomato
¼ cup red bell pepper
1 cup spinach

Juice all of the ingredients. Stir all of the ingredients together and relish every sip!

Heavenly Cantaloupe Cocktail

Serves 3 to 4

2 cantaloupes
½ cup fresh orange juice
2 tsp. fresh lemon juice
½ tsp. lemon zest

Cut the melon in half and remove the seeds. Scoop out the pulp and put it in the blender with the other ingredients. Blend until smooth. Enjoy!

VARIATION: Serve this as a smoothie or as a chilled melon soup. Instead of the cantaloupe, try it with crenshaw, casaba, galia, or honeydew melons.

Beet Veggie Juice

Serves 2 to 3

3 medium beets, quartered
6–8 carrots
6 leaves of romaine lettuce
1 cup fresh spinach
1 cucumber

Juice all of the ingredients and serve immediately. Sip slowly and savor every drop. Adding the juice of a fresh lemon and/or ginger gives it a real zing and adds to the nutritional value.

Rejuvenating Parsley Pear Blend

Serves 2 (makes about 3 cups)

4 ripe pears, cored and quartered
1 bunch curly parsley, stemmed
1 cup water
3–4 ice cubes
Touch of cinnamon

Blend all ingredients until smooth.

VARIATION: If I don't have parsley on hand, I'll substitute romaine lettuce, baby leaf spinach, sunflower sprout greens, or alfalfa or red clover sprouts—or any combination of these green, healthful foods.

Watermelon Ginger Refresher

Serves 3 to 4

5 cups watermelon, seeded and cut into chunks
1½ tbsp. fresh ginger root juice (put through
      your juicer)
1⅓ cups purified water
Fresh mint sprigs

In a blender, blend; then serve.

VARIATION: To create a slushy version, freeze 3 cups of watermelon chunks and blend with the remaining 2 cups of unfrozen watermelon. Pour into glasses that have been chilled in the freezer, and garnish with fresh mint.

Phytonutrient Power Drink

Serves 1 to 2

4 oz. carrot juice
2 oz. celery juice
1 oz. beet juice
1 oz. kale (or watercress) juice
1 oz. broccoli sprout juice
1 apple, cut, cored, and juiced

Stir all ingredients together and enjoy!

VARIATION: I often juice small amounts of lemon, ginger, and parsley to add to the drink.

Smoothies

You'll appreciate your blender after tasting these magnificently colorful ambrosias.

Perfectly Persimmon Smoothie

Serves 2 to 3

2 persimmons
¼ cup pumpkin seeds, soaked for 4 hours and drained
2 dried figs, soaked for 1 hour
1 cup fig-soaking water (or more)
1 banana
⅛ tsp. cinnamon
⅛ tsp. cardamom

Blend and serve.

VARIATION: For some of the liquid, instead of all fig water, substitute coconut water, purified water, or some apple juice.

Chocolate Sweet Potato Smoothie

Serves 2 to 4

2 cups juice (orange, apple, cranberry, almond milk,
     soymilk, or any combination)
1 cup cooked sweet potato or yam flesh
4–5 pitted medjool dates
1 ripe frozen banana
1½ tsp. of pure cocoa (I use 100% organic cocoa powder
     or raw carob powder.)
Dash of cinnamon

Blend until smooth. For a sweeter taste, add a sweetener of your choice (such as more dates, granulized date sugar, pure maple syrup, or stevia). If your banana isn't frozen, add a few ice cubes for more of a shake.

VARIATION: Sometimes I'll eliminate the cocoa and use carob powder and/or fresh ginger, vanilla extract, apple pieces, or the fresh juice of the raw sweet potato so it can be an all-raw tasty treat. I also serve different variations of this "antioxidant" smoothie/shake as a chilled soup.

(For more blender recipes, refer to my website: **www. SusanSmithJones.com**.)

Kiwi Melon Smoothie

Serves 2 to 3

4 kiwis, peeled and cut into chunks
1 cup crenshaw, honeydew, or cantaloupe cubes, frozen
1 cup fresh apple or orange juice
1 tsp. lemon zest

Blend and serve immediately.

VARIATION: Substitute almond or cashew milk, coconut water, or just pure water for the juice. Add some blueberries or raspberries to create a different color and tasty, antioxidant-rich treat.

Glorious Grapefruit Juice/Smoothie

Serves 2 to 3

3 pink or ruby red grapefruits, peeled
2 cups melons (cantaloupe and watermelon are great)
1 cup strawberries

Blend or juice and serve.

VARIATION: Instead of melons, try tangerines and oranges. Substitute blueberries, raspberries, peaches, persimmons, nectarines, cranberries, or cherries for the strawberries. When juicing, I will add some fresh ginger. Sometimes, when making the smoothie version, I'll use organic frozen cherries or other frozen fruit and add a dash of cinnamon.

Cranberry Grape Plunge

Serves 2 to 3

2–3 young coconuts
⅓ cup frozen cranberries
1½ cups seedless grapes (red, green, or
   a combination of both), frozen

Blend the coconut water and the soft coconut meat with the fruit. It produces a wonderful mauve color that's as beautiful to look at as it is scrumptious to taste.

VARIATION: Replace grapes with blueberries, raspberries, blackberries, peaches, cherries, papaya, mango, banana, kiwi, or any combination. Each different fruit boasts a new, resplendent color and a variety of nutrients. I usually use just one fruit so I can enjoy its rich color and sensational taste.

Coconut Fruit Smoothie

Serves 2 to 4

2–3 young coconuts
2 cups frozen fruit

Look for young coconuts at natural-food stores and better grocery and Asian markets. Cut off the top of the coconut with a sharp knife. Pour the coconut water into the blender. Scrape out the coconut meat (soft, gel-like consistency) with a spoon and add this to the mixture. Next, add the frozen fruit and blend until smooth, using extra coconut water or purified water to reach your desired consistency. Pour into glasses and serve.

Strawberry Banana Smoothie

Serves 2 to 3

8 frozen strawberries
1 ripe frozen banana, cut into chunks
¾ cup fresh strawberry juice
½ cup almond or cashew milk (see page 111)
Ice cubes (optional)

Blend all ingredients and serve. If you want it thicker and colder, add ice cubes.

VARIATION: Use coconut water instead of the nut milk and add some mango and papaya for a Tropical Smoothie.

Pomegranate Fruit Smoothie

Serves 2 to 3

1½ cups pomegranate juice
½ cup blueberries, frozen
½ cup strawberries, raspberries, or blackberries (or a
       combination of these berries), frozen
1 banana, peeled (optional)
Ice

Blend to desired consistency and serve.

VARIATION: Substitute frozen peaches, mango, papaya, kiwi, or cherries for the fruit.

Vegetable Salads

These extraordinary salads burst with a rainbow of colors, textures, and tastes.

Crunchy Broccoli Bell Salad

Serves 3 to 5

2 cups broccoli stalks, peeled and diced
3 bell peppers, red, yellow, and orange, de-seeded and
       diced
3 scallions, diced
2 ears of corn, cut off the cob
2 celery stalks, diced
½ cup raisins or goji berries
¼ cup raw sunflower seeds

Combine all of the ingredients and drizzle with your favorite dressing. For a fresh, light taste, try my Fresh & Luscious Lemon Dressing (see page 122).

VARIATION: Replace sunflower seeds with chopped walnuts, almonds, pecans, or cashews. Also try adding diced jicama, asparagus, cauliflower, red onion, and grated carrots.

Savory Cucumber Fennel Salad

Serves 2 to 4

2 cucumbers, chopped
1 fennel bulb
1 small red onion, diced
2 vine-ripened tomatoes, chopped
½ cup flat-leaf parsley, chopped
Hearts of romaine

Cut off the bottom of the fennel. Shave off thin slices and then julienne the thin slices. Mix all the ingredients and dress with Fresh & Luscious Lemon Dressing (page 122) or Orange Balsamic Vinaigrette (page 123). Place on a bed of romaine hearts.

VARIATION: Place the salad on a bed of fresh spinach and arugala. Add your favorite chopped herbs. Use chopped green onions or shallots instead of the red onion. Substitute cherry tomatoes (cut in half) in different colors for the bigger tomatoes.

Corny Onion Salad

Serves 3 to 4

1 red onion, diced
2 sweet onions, diced
1 shallot, diced
5 green onions, chopped
4 ears of corn, cut off the cob
1 cucumber, diced
½ cup cherry tomatoes, halved
¼ cup finely chopped parsley
Fresh mixed greens such as mescaline, spinach,
**   arugala, and romaine**

Mix all ingredients (except the greens) together with your favorite dressing. Serve on top of the greens. I like this with the Fresh & Luscious Lemon (page 122), Grapefruit Tahini (page 122), or Orange Balsamic Vinaigrette dressings (page 123). The parsley will help sweeten your breath.

Fruit Salads

For some great snacks and exotic mealtime extravaganzas, try these sweet treats.

Banana Bites

Serves 3 to 4

3 large bananas, peeled
21 pecans
21 raisins or goji berries
3–4 butterhead lettuce leaves

Cut the bananas into 20 equal rounds—about 7 slices for each banana. Press one raisin or goji berry down into the top of each banana slice, deep enough to create a flat top. Place a pecan on each banana round, place the rounds in lettuce leaves, and see how quickly they disappear.

VARIATION: Use walnut halves instead of pecans. Sprinkle some freshly grated coconut meat on the banana round before topping it with a nut. Try macadamia nuts instead of pecans. Sprinkle the banana rounds with a dash of cinnamon before topping with the nut.

Citrus Cinnamon Delight

Serves 1 or more

Romaine lettuce, cut up
Pink or red grapefruit slices, diced
Orange slices, diced
Kiwi slices, diced
Pinch of cinnamon

I didn't put amounts for these ingredients because it depends on how hungry I am! Arrange a generous amount of cut-up lettuce on a plate. Place diced fruit on top of the lettuce. Sprinkle cinnamon over the fruit. This is one of my favorite breakfast meals.

VARIATION: Substitute any of your favorite fruits.

Dressings & Dips

Treat yourself and your guests to these scrumptiously delicious dressings.

Grapefruit Tahini Dressing

Makes about 1 cup

½ cup tahini (I use raw tahini)
3 tbsp. fresh grapefruit juice
1 tbsp. fresh lemon juice
⅓ cup water (or more)
Celtic sea salt to taste (optional)

Blend all of the ingredients until smooth. Add more water if you prefer a thinner consistency. Use within 5 days. Keep refrigerated.

VARIATION: Use all lemon juice to replace the grapefruit juice and you have Lemon Tahini Dressing. Add some minced garlic, chopped parsley, and dashes of cumin and turmeric, and blend.

Fresh & Luscious Lemon Dressing

Makes about ¾ cup

3 lemons (a little over ⅓ cup)
½ cup extra-virgin, cold-pressed fresh olive oil
1–2 cloves garlic (optional)
Celtic sea salt to taste (optional)

Juice the lemons in a citrus juicer or with a citrus reamer. Press the garlic in a bowl, and pour in the juice. Whisk in the olive oil. Salt to taste (optional). Keep refrigerated.

VARIATION: Substitute ½ cup or less of fresh grapefruit juice instead of lemon juice; replace some or all of the olive oil with flaxseed oil. Blend in a tomato to this recipe to make it more of a fresh-style dressing. Add your favorite herbs such as parsley, oregano, thyme, basil, or tarragon.

Orange Balsamic Vinaigrette

Makes about ½ cup

3 tbsp. extra-virgin, cold-pressed olive oil
1 tbsp. fresh orange juice
1 tbsp. organic balsamic vinegar
1 tsp. Dijon mustard
1 tsp. zest from an organic orange
¼ tsp. Celtic sea salt (optional)

In a blender, jar, or small bowl, thoroughly combine all the ingredients. Just before serving, drizzle over your salad and toss.

Groovy Guacamole

Makes about 3 cups

2 avocados, peeled and seeds removed
½ medium serrano chili, de-seeded and diced
1 red onion, diced
1–2 ears of corn, cut off the cob
1 clove garlic
2 tomatoes, quartered
¼ cup cilantro, chopped (optional)
1 tbsp. fresh lemon or lime juice
Celtic sea salt to taste (optional)

Chop the garlic and chili. Put all the ingredients in a food processor or blender and pulse until desired consistency. For chunkier guacamole, don't process one of the avocados—instead, dice it and mix it in afterwards.

VARIATION: Add the juice of an orange to the ingredients. Leave out the tomatoes and add a cup of chopped spinach or watercress. Add some cumin powder. Add coriander, basil, or mint to the ingredients before blending. Add a banana to the ingredients before blending to give it a sweet taste.

Sensational Salsa

Makes about 2½ cups

1¾ cups tomatoes, diced
2 tbsp. onion, finely diced
1 tbsp. red bell pepper, finely diced
1 tbsp. yellow bell pepper, finely diced
1 jalapeño chili, de-seeded, white rib removed, minced
1 tbsp. fresh cilantro, chopped
1 tsp. or more garlic, minced or pressed
⅛ tsp. ginger, minced (optional)
2 tbsp. fresh lime juice
Celtic sea salt to taste (optional)

In a food processor or blender, pulse until desired consistency, or simply mix all of the ingredients thoroughly in a bowl. Refrigerate until ready to serve.

VARIATION: For Corn Salsa, add ½ cup corn kernels. For Mango Salsa, add ½ cup diced mango. For Avocado Salsa, add ½ cup to ¾ cup diced avocado. For a sweeter salsa, add ⅓ cup raisins. For Jicama Salsa, add ½ cup diced jicama.

RECIPE TIPS: In addition to using salsa as a dip for tortilla chips, raw vegetables, or a variety of Mexican dishes, try it on brown rice, millet, or quinoa, or as a topping on baked potatoes or steamed vegetables, or wrapped in lettuce leaves and nori sheets with some avocado slices, grated carrots, and other vegetables.

Tahini Salsa Dressing

Makes 2 cups

1 cup Grapefruit or Lemon Tahini Dressing *(see page 122)*
1 cup Sensational Salsa *(see above)*

In a medium bowl, combine the dressing and the salsa thoroughly, and serve. Store in the refrigerator for up to 5 days. This dressing gives any salad a Tex-Mex flavor and also is great on baked potatoes, steamed vegetables, or as a dip.

Spicy Sprouted Hummus

Serves 4

3 cups sprouted chickpeas
¼ –½ cup raw tahini
¼ cup freshly squeezed lemon juice
1–2 cloves garlic, peeled and minced
⅛ –¼ tsp. cayenne pepper
1 tsp. kelp powder
¼ cup purified water or fresh celery juice to reach
    desired consistency (add more if needed)
Paprika

In a blender or food processor, purée the sprouted chickpeas with the water or celery juice. Add the remaining ingredients and blend until smooth. Place the hummus in a bowl and sprinkle with cayenne or paprika, depending on your "hot" taste.

VARIATION: For an eye-catching change, add ½ cup chopped parsley or cilantro or a combination of both for a green hummus. I also make hummus with 2 cups of almonds, soaked overnight, then rinsed, in place of the beans, and add extra lemon juice and tahini to create the desired consistency and taste. It's also delicious with chopped fresh spearmint.

RECIPE TIPS: This hummus recipe really shows the advantages of the Total Blender. I burned out several other blenders before I found it. Garbanzo beans (a.k.a. chickpeas) are quick and easy to sprout. Soak (germinate) overnight for 8 hours in a covered glass container with purified water. Drain and sprout for one day (12 hours). The best flavor comes from using garbanzos that have been sprouted for at least one day. When I've been in a hurry, I've used soaked chickpeas without sprouting them. I also use and recommend heirloom-quality chickpeas that are black and dark brown for a beautiful eye-treat.

Mellow Mushroom Gravy

Makes about 3 cups

2 cups Portobello mushrooms
1 small red onion
6 stalks of celery
1 lemon
1 clove garlic
½ tsp. paprika

Juice the celery stalks and lemon. Put in a bowl with the paprika. Finely chop the mushrooms, garlic, and onions. Add to the juice mixture and marinade 1 to 6 hours—the longer the better. Add all of the ingredients to a blender and blend. If you want it warmed, stir over a low flame. Do not overheat.

Cranberry Pineapple Relish

Makes about 5 cups

1 bag cranberries (12-oz. bag or ¾ lb.)
1 pineapple, cut into chunks
¾ cup pecans
Pinch of stevia, to taste

In a food processor or blender, pulse (chop) for a few seconds. Keep it chunky and not puréed.

VARIATION: Use walnuts in place of the pecans. Stir in some fresh blueberries or raspberries or some freshly grated coconut meat to mingle with the cranberries. Add a dash of cinnamon and freshly grated nutmeg. Makes a great holiday cranberry relish too.

Fruit & Nut Toppings

These unique taste treats add flair and style to your favorite foods.

Vanilla Orange Cream

Makes about 1½ cups

2 oranges, juiced
1 cup macadamia nuts (walnuts, Brazil nuts, cashews,
    or other nuts also can be used)
¼ tsp. lemon zest
2 inches fresh vanilla pod
1 tbsp. fresh lime juice

In a blender or food processor, blend all of the ingredients. If you desire it thicker, add more nuts. For a thinner version, add more orange juice. It stays fresh for a couple of days in the refrigerator.

Omega-3 Walnut-Flax Topping

Makes about ⅔ cup

⅓ cup organic golden flaxseed, ground
⅓ cup organic walnuts, ground

Grind each separately or together and sprinkle over your favorite foods.

VARIATION: As a topping for cereals, mix in some cinnamon. As a topping for grains and vegetables, mix in some cumin or coriander. For a sweet and savory blend, mix in some cardamom. For a spicy note, mix in some cayenne and ground ginger.

Fabulous Fig Sauce

Serves 1 or more

Dried Mission figs
Purified water

Soak figs in water until soft. Blend figs, adding enough of the remaining liquid to form a delicious, chocolate-like sauce to serve on fruits such as strawberries or apple wedges.

VARIATION: For a thicker sauce, use less liquid; for a thinner sauce, add more rehydrating liquid. Experiment with your own measurements. A pinch of cinnamon or nutmeg is a tasty addition too.

Pear Cashew Cream Topping

Makes about 3 cups

2 pears
2 cups purified water
1 cup raw cashews
⅛ tsp. cinnamon

Peel and dice pears. In a blender or food processor, blend together all ingredients until smooth. Chill. This is a superb dressing for fruit or other desserts. This makes a delicious dip for strawberries, quartered apples, or other fresh fruit.

VARIATION: Substitute coconut water for some or all of the purified water. Add some freshly grated nutmeg (use a Microplane). A couple of chopped mint leaves add a nice touch too.

Soups and Bisque

These savory soups can enhance any meal or be the perfect snack.

Sweet Pepper & Almond Soup

Serves 4

2 cups almond milk
4 red, yellow, or orange sweet peppers, de-seeded
4 sun-dried tomatoes, soaked
½ cup fresh coriander, finely chopped
1 small onion, peeled and finely chopped
Pinch each of cumin, turmeric, and coriander powder

Separate the fresh coriander, two teaspoons of onion, and one sun-dried tomato. Place all other ingredients in the blender and blend thoroughly. You can strain the soup before serving, if desired. Add the chopped coriander and mix well. Pour into serving bowls. Dice the remaining sun-dried tomato, mix with the remaining onion, and top the soup with this mixture.

Chilled Berry Blueberry Soup

Serves 3 to 4

3 cups fresh blueberries
2 cups fresh raspberries or strawberries or combination
of both
2 cups cashew milk *(see Almond Milk recipe on page 111)*
1 tsp. fresh mint leaves, chopped
Dash of cinnamon

Put all ingredients in the blender and blend to desired consistency. Pour into serving bowls and garnish with a fresh mint leaf.

VARIATION: If you want your soup thicker, blend in a few whole cashews or add more fruit. Try the recipe with blueberries, blackberries, and cranberries and, instead of two cups of cashew milk, substitute one cup of fresh coconut water.

Spicy Sweet Potato Bisque

Serves 3 to 4

4 sweet potatoes, juiced
2 cups Sesame Milk (see page 110)
1 avocado, de-seeded, peeled, and cubed
⅓ cup cashews, soaked for 2 hours and drained
½ cup sweet onion, finely diced
¼ cup chives, finely chopped
1 tbsp. coconut butter
¼ tsp. allspice
¼ tsp. cardamom
¼ tsp. mace
Celtic sea salt to taste (optional)

Blend the sweet potato juice, sesame milk, avocado, and spices until smooth. Pour into serving bowls and stir in the desired amount of onion and chives.

Golden Gazpacho Soup

Serves 4

10 ripe yellow or red tomatoes (I use heirloom when
    available)
1 cup onion, diced
2 red peppers, one juiced and one diced (or half red
    and half orange)
1 large cucumber, half-diced and half-juiced
1 medium red chili, finely chopped
2 stalks celery, juiced
⅓ lemon, juiced
1 clove garlic, finely chopped
Bunch of chives and coriander

Juice 8 of the tomatoes, half of the cucumber, the lemon, celery, and half of the red pepper. Finely chop the rest of the ingredients and mix them together. Garnish with chopped herbs and a dollop of Vanilla Orange Cream (see page 127).

VII

MOTIVATIONAL TOOLS

SETTING UP YOUR HEALTHY KITCHEN

When planning your grocery lists, whenever possible, go for organic foods. If your local supermarket is short on their organic selection, make friends with the produce manager. The more people who request organic foods—not only fresh fruits and vegetables, but also legumes, seeds, nuts, teas, and whole grains—the greater the chance the store buyer will accommodate. They want to keep their customers happy.

I frequent several local natural-food stores as well as the variety of farmers' markets in my area, so it's not difficult for me to eat a predominantly organic diet. However, if you're not having any luck with your supermarket produce manager, if you don't have any natural-food stores or farmers' markets in your area, and if you can't grow the produce yourself in your yard or container pots, there are always mail-order catalogs that will deliver right to your door. For convenience and price discounts, I sometimes purchase legumes, grains, dried mushrooms, and dried fruit, along with organic teas, seeds, and nuts, through mail-order.

It's more difficult to purchase fresh produce through the mail because of the "freshness" factor. When selecting fruits and vegetables in your local market, try to find the freshest foods available. And, as I mentioned earlier in the book, if you just can't get organic produce, wash your commercially grown foods well and enjoy them. I'm going to let you in on an important, but little-discussed, secret. Every time you buy produce that isn't certified organic—that is, grown without conventional pesticides and fertilizers—you're bringing home *potentially* harmful chemicals. But these chemicals have not been proven to be even remotely as harmful to health as eating the highly processed, denatured, high-salt-, high-fat-, and high-cholesterol-laden standard American diet. Plus, while organic produce is higher in nutrients than conventionally grown produce, the differences typically are not dramatic. So don't make the mistake of sticking with an unhealthful, conventional diet just because you can't find organic varieties of the NATUREFOODS I have been championing. If cost is a factor, and you simply can't afford to buy all organic food, splurge first on lettuce and other leafy greens, since they have the largest surface area on which the chemicals can adhere.

Thankfully, not all conventionally grown fruits and vegetables are vulnerable. Which should you be most careful about? The Environmental Working Group, a leading American consumer watchdog organization, has come up with lists of the best and worst produce in pesticide residue.

Take these following fruit and vegetable lists with you when shopping. Fruits highest in pesticides: *Apples, cherries, imported grapes, nectarines, peaches, pears, raspberries, strawberries.* Fruits lowest in pesticides: *avocados, bananas, blueberries, grapefruit, kiwi fruit, mangoes, papayas, pineapples, plantains, plums, watermelons.* Vegetables highest in pesticides: *Bell peppers, celery, hot peppers, potatoes, spinach.* Vegetables lowest in pesticides: *Asparagus and broccoli.*

As you get more interested in where and how your food is grown, you will learn what foods can be grown organically or near-organically in your area. Remember, the purchase and application of farm chemicals cost money, so farmers don't use them on crops just for the fun of it. In the right place, in the right season, many crops for local consumption can be grown with little or no chemical application.

KITCHEN TOOLS

As I mentioned earlier, no matter how much you enjoy meal preparation, it helps to have available a few culinary tools that make it easier and faster to prepare healthful meals. I'll briefly mention my must-have list again—various knives, whisks, a colander and sieve, mixing bowls and spoons, a salad spinner, a couple of Microplanes, nonstick pans, sprouting utensils, a citrus reamer, a garlic press, cutting boards, cookware, a nut/seed grinder, a citrus juicer, a food processor, and Champion juicer. Your list may vary, but a few important appliances really need to become part of everyone's healthy kitchen.

BLENDER

Indispensable in my healthy kitchen, cuisine classes around the country, and private culinary instruction and adventures, the blender is a miracle to me. As I mentioned, I use mine several times every day to make soups, smoothies, vegetarian "cheese" sauces, dressings, nut milks, "ice cream", purées, and nut butters. Put simply, if there was only one kitchen appliance I could have, it would be a blender. Of course, like everything else, there are many different types of blenders and prices, and I've tried them all.

The grand prix of all blenders is made by Blendtec®. The price is higher than the regular department-store blenders—and it's well worth it! This machine has no problem chopping ice or blending nuts and seeds into delicious butters. Less expensive machines are great for smoothies, soups, and dressings, but you will have to be careful not to burn out the motor when making nut cheeses or nut butters. Blendtec makes two blenders for home use. I use the Total Blender at home and also take it with me on the road to use in my workshops and healthful-food-preparation classes. Their Connoisseur is the same blender quality, but the difference is that it can be installed right in your kitchen counter (better for home owners, not renters), so it's convenient and takes up less space. The same engineering genius goes into both blenders. The computer-controlled blend cycles make perfect drinks and recipes with one-touch operation. No old-fashioned knobs, switches, or dials to wear out. Solid-state electronics and a sleek touchpad ensure long life and dependable performance. No other blender offers the power, ease of operation, and state-of-the-art engineering. The half-gallon-capacity jar is lightweight and easy to clean. A powerful 3-peak horsepower motor makes any blending operation a joy. Both the Total Blender and the Connoisseur are extraordinary blenders and my pick for everyone who has a kitchen. They will become your best friends in the kitchen and improve your healthful-meal preparation immeasurably. You'll be able to create gourmet meals in seconds.

Here's a tip for cleaning your blender. Fill it halfway with warm water and a couple of drops of liquid dishwashing soap. With the lid in place, turn it on high for about 30 seconds. Rinse it out and, voilà, it's clean and ready for your next use.

For more information or to order the Total Blender or the Kitchen Mill, please visit: **www.SusanSmithJones.com**, click on *Susan's Favorite Products*, and then click on *Blendtec home*.

IONIZER PLUS

As mentioned on pages 63–65, when we alkalize our bodies, we maximize our health. The Ionizer Plus first filters the tap water to remove contaminants, chlorine, chemicals, taste, and smell. Then the water is treated with ultraviolet light for disinfection. Next it enters an electrolysis chamber where it is treated with a precise direct current that divides it into two distinctly different types of water, *alkali-ion* and *acidic-ion*. In the process, the molecular cluster (size) of both types of water is broken down from 10 to 12 molecules per cluster to 4 to 6 molecules. The resulting water permeates the body quickly and efficiently. Alkaline ion water is not only smaller but also contains more calcium, magnesium, and potassium ions. These naturally occurring water-soluble minerals are alkaline by nature and thus increase the alkalinity (pH) of this water. Acidic-ion water is slightly astringent, and its penetrating capability and lower pH have a healthy effect on your skin and hair. The water from the Ionizer Plus is also perfect to use with the Activated Air machine described on the next page. For more information, please refer to my website and click on *Susan's Favorite Products*. You can also call 00-1-800-794-5355 or visit: **www.hightechhealth.com**.

ACTIVATED AIR

Here's something wonderful that I enjoy using in my kitchen when preparing meals or sitting at the kitchen table with a cup of fresh juice or tea and a good book, as well as in other rooms of my home. One of my favorite health-promoting products, Activated Air is a stellar breathing therapy developed by European scientists to combat free radicals, help keep our cellular energy production in top shape, and best protect us against illness and the effects of aging. Also, if you're interested in losing weight, you'll want to get an Activated Air device. With maximized oxygen uptake, you burn fat more easily as your body's fuel source. In other words, you will have an easier time losing weight, especially when combined with an optimum diet (described in this book) and regular exercise. Even your pets can reap the benefits of this simple, superlative machine. This inimitable device has made a profound, positive difference in my life, as well as in the lives of many of my clients and friends. Simple to use, it takes just 20 minutes, three times a week, and you'll see a difference too. I use mine daily when watching TV, stretching, meditating, or working at my desk or computer. Visit: **www.SusanSmithJones.com**, click on *Susan's Favorite Products,* and read my article, "A Healthier Life Is Just a Few Breaths Away." For more information or to order an Activated Air machine, please call: 00-1-877-571-9206 or visit: **www.eng3corp.com**.

CHAMPION 2000+ JUICER

There are many fruit and vegetable juicers on the market, but for the highest quality, I always recommend the Champion 2000+ Juicer. It makes preparing fresh, wholesome fruit and vegetable juices a joy.

One of the best known and most popular worldwide, the Champion 2000+ Juicer includes a number of features that bring the power and durability of commercial juicers directly to your kitchen countertop. Delicious fruit and vegetable juices of the highest quality have never been easier to prepare. Juice from the

Champion 2000+ is darker, richer in color, and contains more of the nutrients you desire than that produced by other juicers.

Two more of the many reasons that I choose to use the Champion 2000+ is because it is easy to clean, and it does so much more than juicing. In fact, it's the ultimate multitask, culinary machine. I also use it to make fruit sauces and purées; sorbets, sherbets, and "ice cream" (from frozen fruit); baby foods; and creamy nut butters. The Champion 2000+ also functions as a grain mill, allowing you to quickly and easily prepare healthy, hearty whole grains.

For more information or to order a Champion 2000+ Juicer, call: 00 1 866 WE JUICE (935-8423) or visit: **www.championjuicer.com**.

* * *

AFTERWORD

Thoughts to Inspire as You Transform Your Life!

Here are some of my favorite quotes. They've inspired me over the years, and I hope that they will inspire you too. At birth, each of us is given the divine gift of *laziness*—the extremely important survival instinct to conserve energy. This conservation-of-energy instinct helped us survive in the millennia before the wheel, running water, electricity, and the disposable diaper. Of necessity, we mastered the art of weighing the risks and efforts required to attempt something against the potential benefits of succeeding at it. In simple terms, we learned not to "waste our valuable time or energy" unless we thought it was "worth it".

Changing your diet, making new shopping and kitchen habits, and learning how to be the "new you" in environments that are not always supportive can require considerable effort. Don't let your instinctive drive to conserve energy interfere with your desire to be all you can be. The following quotes can help you focus on the deeper meanings of life and the joys of dedicating your life to them.

George Bernard Shaw, never a man to mince words, put it this way:

> "This is the true joy in life, the being used for a purpose recognized by yourself as a mighty one . . . being a force of Nature instead of a feverish selfish little clod of ailments and grievances complaining that the world will not devote itself to making you happy."

Best wishes as you begin your personal journey to health and happiness!

"Be transformed by the renewing of your mind."
—Romans 12:2

"You can accomplish anything if you do not accept limitations . . .
whatever you make up your mind to do, you can do."
—Paramahansa Yogananda

"Oh, while I live to be the ruler of life, not a slave,
to meet life as a powerful conqueror,
and nothing exterior to me shall ever take command of me."
—Walt Whitman

"What lies behind us and what lies before us are small matters
compared to what lies within us."
—Ralph Waldo Emerson

"We need to find God, and He cannot be found in noise and restlessness.
God is the friend of silence."
—Mother Teresa

"Delight yourself in the Lord, and He shall give you the desires of your heart."
—Psalm 37:4

"Wake at dawn with a winged heart, and give thanks for another day of loving."
—Kahlil Gibran

"Of course I love everyone I meet. How could I fail to?
Within everyone is the spark of God.
I am not concerned with racial or ethnic background or the color of one's skin;
all people look to me like shining lights!"
—Peace Pilgrim

"Eat to live, don't live to eat; many dishes, many diseases."
—**Benjamin Franklin**

"Your health, happiness, and the future of life on Earth
are rarely so much in your own hands as when you sit down to eat."
—**John Robbins**

"It is a great relief when for a few moments in the day
we can retire to our chamber to be completely true to ourselves.
It leavens the rest of our hours."
—**Henry David Thoreau**

"Remember always that you not only have the right to be an individual,
you also have an obligation to be one."
—**Eleanor Roosevelt**

"I submit that scientists have not yet explored the hidden possibilities
of the innumerable seeds, leaves, and fruits
for giving the fullest possible nutrition to mankind."
—**Mahatma Gandhi**

"There is absolutely no substitute for greens in the diet!
If you refuse to eat these 'sunlight energy' foods,
you are depriving yourself, to a large degree,
of the very essence of life."
—**H. E. Kirschner, MD**

"If doctors, with all of their knowledge of the human body,
would merely become familiar with the principles of health and
the simple Natural Laws that God established, and share them,
they would be performing the greatest humanitarian service
to mankind this world has ever known."
—**Dr. George H. Malkmus**

*"Hope is the thing with feathers
That perches in the soul
And sings the tune with words
And never stops at all."*
—Emily Dickinson

*"No matter what will be said and done,
preserve your calm immovably;
and to every obstacle, oppose patience,
perseverance, and soothing language."*
—Thomas Jefferson

*"If we did all the things we are capable of doing,
we would literally astound ourselves."*
—Thomas Alva Edison

*"Sometimes you can't see yourself clearly
until you see yourself through the eyes of others."*
—Ellen DeGeneres

*"If you look at what you have in life,
you'll always have more.
If you look at what you don't have,
you'll never have enough."*
—Oprah Winfrey

* * *

VIII

RESOURCES

RECOMMENDED READING, REFERENCES & OTHER RESOURCES

Alt, Carol. *Eating in the Raw.* New York: Clarkson Potter Publishers, 2004.

American Vegan Society. www.americanvegan.org

Back to the Garden. www.hacres.com

Barnard, Neal D., MD. *Breaking the Food Seduction: The Hidden Reasons Behind Food Cravings—and 7 Steps to End Them Naturally.* New York: St. Martin's Press, 2003.

Baroody, Theodore A., PhD. *Alkalize or Die.* Waynesville: Holographic Health Press, 8th Printing, 2002.

Campbell, T. Colin, PhD, with Campbell, Thomas M., II. *The China Study: Startling Implications for Diet, Weight Loss, and Long-Term Health.* Dallas: Benbella Books, 2005.

Cousens, Gabriel, MD. *Conscious Eating.* Berkeley: North Atlantic Publishing, 2005.

———. *Rainbow Green Live-Food Cuisine.* Berkeley: North Atlantic Publishing, 2004.

Fife, Bruce, CN, ND. *The Coconut Oil Miracle.* New York: Avery, 2004.

Fuhrman, Joel, MD. *Cholesterol Protection For Life.* Flemington, NJ: Gift of Health Press, 2006.

———. *Disease-Proof Your Child—Feeding Kids Right.* New York: St. Martin's Press, 2005.

Good Medicine. www.pcrm.org

Haas, Elson M., MD. *Staying Healthy with Nutrition.* Berkeley: Celestial Arts, 2006. (New Edition)

Hay, Louise. *Heal Your Body.* Carlsbad: Hay House, 2001.

————. *Power Thoughts: 365 Daily Affirmations.* Carlsbad: Hay House, 2005.

————. *You Can Heal Your Life.* Carlsbad: Hay House, 2003.

Health Science. www.healthscience.org

Heber, David, MD, PhD. *What Color Is Your Diet?* New York: Regan Books, 2001.

Jones, Susan Smith, PhD. *The Healing Power of NatureFoods: Volume 2.* Carlsbad: Hay House. (Look for this in 2008.)

————. *The Healing Power of NatureFoods: Volume 3.* Carlsbad: Hay House. (Look for this in 2009.)

————. *Wired to Meditate, Celebrate Life!, Choose to Live Peacefully,* and other audio programs. (www.SusanSmithJones.com)

Jones, Susan Smith, and Warren, Dianne. *Vegetable Soup/The Fruit Bowl.* Sarasota: Oasis Publishing, 2007 (4th printing). (www.SusanSmithJones.com)

Joseph, James A., Nadeau, Daniel A., and Underwood, Anne. *The Color Code.* New York: Hyperion, 2002.

Kenney, Mathew, and Melngailis, Sarma. *Raw Food/Real Food.* NewYork: ReganBooks, 2005.

Khalsa, Dharma Singh, MD. *Food as Medicine.* New York: Atria Books, 2003.

Klein, David. *Self Healing Colitis & Crohn's.* Sebastopol: Living Nutrition Publications, 2005.

Living Nutrition. www.livingnutrition.com

Malkmus, George H. *God's Way to Ultimate Health.* Shelby: Hallelujah Acres Publishing, 20th Printing, 2004.

Mars, Brigitte. *Rawsome!* North Bergen: Basic Health Publications, 2004.

Meyerowitz, Steve. *The Organic Food Guide.* Guilford: The Globe Pequot Press, 2004.

————. *Power Juices Super Drinks.* New York: Kensington Books, 2000.

Moran, Victoria. *Fat, Broke & Lonely: The Stupid Lie That Runs Your Life and 5 Smart Strategies for Breaking Free.* San Francisco: HarperSanFrancisco, 2007.

National Health Association. www.healthscience.org

North American Vegetarian Society. www.NAVS-online.org

Nungesser, Charles, and Nungesser, George. *How We All Went RAW.* Mesa: In the Beginning Health Ministry, 2004.

Nutrition Action Health Letter. www.cspinet.org

Onstad, Dianne. *Whole Foods Companion: A Guide for Adventurous Cooks, Curious Shoppers, and Lovers of Natural Foods.* White River Junction, VT: Chelsea Green Publishing, 2005.

Ornish, Dean, MD. *Dr. Dean Ornish's Program for Reversing Heart Disease.* New York: Ballantine Books, 2005.

Pitchford, Paul. *Healing with Whole Foods.* Berkeley: North Atlantic Books, 2002.

Pratt, Steven, MD, and Matthews, Kathy. *SuperFoods Rx.* New York: HarperCollins Publishers, 2004.

Reader's Digest. *Foods That Harm, Foods That Heal.* Pleasantville: Reader's Digest, 2004.

Rhio. *Hooked on Raw: Rejuvenate Your Body and Soul with Nature's Living Foods.* New York: Beso Entertainment, 2000.

Rose, Natalia. *The Raw Food Detox Diet.* New York: ReganBooks, 2005.

Schlosser, Eric. *Chew on This: Everything You Don't Want to Know about Fast Food.* New York: Houghton Mifflin Co., 2006.

Smith, Lendon H., MD. *Happiness Is a Healthy Life.* New York: McGraw Hill, 1999.

Warren, Dianne. *Family Meals/Comidas en Familia.* Sarasota: Oasis Publications, 2007. www.fitness4kidz.com

_____. *Look at Me/Mirame.* Sarasota: Oasis Publications, 2006. www.fitness4kidz.com

Wood, Rebecca. *The New Whole Foods Encyclopedia.* New York: Penguin Books, 1999.

Yeager, Selene, and the Editors of *Prevention* Health Books. *The Doctors Book of Food Remedies.* Emmanus, PA: Rodale, 1998.

MORE OF MY FAVORITE HEALTH-PROMOTING PRODUCTS

- *Activated Air:* **www.eng3corp.com**, 001-877-571-9206

- *Ionizer Plus:* **www.hightechhealth.com**, 001-800-794-5355

- *Health Mate Infrared Saunas:* **www.healthmatesauna.com**, 001-800-946-60010

- *Excalibur Food Dehydration:* **www.drying123.com**, 001-800-875-4254

- *AlkaLife:* **www.alkalife.com**, 001-888-261-0870, 001-305-235-5120

- *Living Harvest:* **www.livingharvest.com**

- *Age in Reverse:* **www.ageeasy.com**, 001-888-Age-Easy

- *Lydia's Organics:* **www.lydiasorganics.com**

- *Food-Based Protein Energizer Powder:* **www.rainbowlight.com**

- *LaraBar:* **www.larabar.com**

- *Kyolic Aged Garlic Extract:* **www.kyolic.com**

* * *

Books & Audio Programs
by Susan Smith Jones

Vegetable Soup/The Fruit Bowl

Vegetable Soup—The Nutritional ABC's and *The Fruit Bowl—A Contest Among the Fruit,* co-authored by Dianne Warren, are two picture books in one, teaching nutrition for young children. Via beautiful four-color illustrations and rhyming verse, the text introduces children to the connection between what they eat and how they look, feel, and perform. In addition to teaching about fresh whole foods—how they grow and why they are good—the book helps develop math and reading skills as the child becomes an active participant in the reading process. David Klein, publisher of *Living Nutrition,* praised it as "a wonderful children's book introducing the nutritional ABC's (apples-broccoli-spinach) of whole foods!"

Choose to Live Peacefully—Audio Book (3 tapes)

In this celebrated audio book, Susan examines the many facets that comprise a peaceful, balanced life, including how to take loving care of ourselves, restore youthful vitality and create radiant health, connect with our inherent intuitive nature, and bring sacred spirituality into our daily lives with ease and grace. In simple yet inspiring language, Susan offers an empowering 40-day, easy-to-follow program on how to live more fully—healthfully, joyfully, passionately, and peacefully.

Wired to Meditate—Audio Book (2 tapes)

In this delightful audio book, Susan shares her fresh, dynamic approach to unleashing your inner joy and developing your fullest potential. You'll learn how to use meditation and mind power to reduce stress and fulfill your dreams, neutralize negative emotions, make peace and prosperity your constant companions, release fear and awaken to your best self, harness your empowered inner presence to heal your body, practice simple breathing techniques that will lift your spirit and help you feel more serene, and much more.

Celebrate Life!—7-Tape Audio Program

From this enthralling and motivating series, you'll understand how to enrich and transform the quality of your life and experience greater health and more joy, peace, and love than ever before. Some of the topics covered include how to reverse the aging process; create a fit, healthy body; release bad habits; detoxify and rejuvenate your body; stay motivated to exercise; overcome stress, fatigue, and depression; build loving, supportive relationships; and live more from inner guidance. This set includes 7 motivational presentations, 6 guided meditations, and a flyer with Susan's favorite positive affirmations to guide you on creating the life you desire and deserve.

Live Recordings

The following 2-tape albums were recorded live at Susan's popular series of Healthy Living seminars presented worldwide.

- *Choose to Live a Balanced Life:*
  Learn How to Be Healthy, Live Peacefully, and Celebrate Life

- *Make Your Life a Great Adventure:*
  Living an Ordinary Life in an Extraordinary Way

- *A Fresh Start:*
  Rejuvenate Your Body and Life Each and Every Day

* * *

To order Susan's books and audio programs, call: 00 1 800-843-5743
or visit her website:

www.SusanSmithJones.com

(You also can order *Vegetable Soup/The Fruit Bowl* by calling: 00 1 800-915-9355.)

Ongoing Education & Support

"Be the change you wish to see in the world . . ."
— **Gandhi**

I encourage you to join the National Health Association (NHA). Founded in 1948, their mission is to educate and empower individuals to understand that health results from healthful living. They recognize the integration of all aspects of health—personal, environmental, and social. They communicate the benefits of a plant-based, whole-foods diet; exercise and rest; a healthy environment; and psychological wellbeing. When you become a member, you can take advantage of discounts on their conferences, seminars, books, and tapes, and receive their award-winning quarterly magazine, *Health Science. Health Science* focuses on "Health through Healthful Living" and has readers in almost 50 countries.

Membership is only $35 for one year in Canada and USA ($65 for two years) or $55 for one year in all other countries ($95 for two years), payable in an International Money Order in U.S. currency, check drawn on a U.S. bank, or credit card. I've been a member for 35 years, have attended dozens of conferences, purchased countless books and audio programs, written for their magazine, and gained a wealth of valuable knowledge that helps keep me radiantly healthy and disease-free. Becoming a member of NHA is one of the best health gifts you can give yourself, and can be done quickly and easily on their Website: **www.healthscience.org** or by calling: 00 1 813 855-6607.

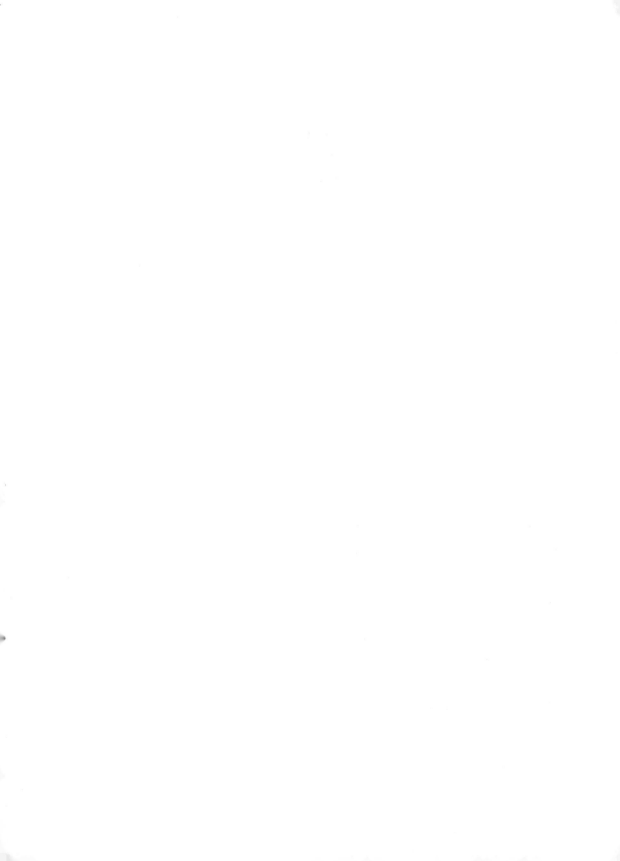

9 Tips to Create More Joy & Less Stress

1. Take time to nourish your body and soul with a balanced diet of wholesome natural foods. Choose from a wide variety of colorful foods as close to the way nature made them as possible. Vary your diet daily, and strive for as much fresh, raw food as possible. Living foods increase energy, restore youthful vitality, and promote radiant health.

2. Drink at least 8 glasses of water daily. Lack of moisture in faces creates wrinkles the way lack of moisture in plums creates prunes. Drinking ample water is necessary to lubricate your joints, feed your cells, and keep your skin—that constantly loses moisture to the environment—clear, soft, and youthful. Pure water fosters vitality.

3. Eat only as much as needed and not much after nightfall—within two to three hours before sleep. Grazing on *smaller* meals and snacks more frequently throughout the day—every two to three hours—stokes metabolism, stabilizes blood sugar, and helps reduce cholesterol and unhealthful habits of overeating. It's prudent to plan meals so you won't get famished.

4. Exercise regularly and find a balance of strengthening, stretching, and aerobic activities. Make your program a top priority in your life, a non-negotiable activity, and stay committed to it! There is nothing that will benefit you more in terms of being happy, disease-free, vibrantly youthful, and

energetic than a regular fitness program. Whenever possible, exercise outdoors in a natural, beautiful environment.

5. Sleep well—at least seven to eight hours nightly. Consistent lack of sleep leads to many health problems, including wrinkles, depression, weight gain and aging, low or no libido, toxic build-up, irritability and impatience, memory loss, lethargy, relationship problems, and accidents. Refrain from watching bedtime TV news. Make your bedroom an exquisite, peaceful sanctuary. Put three drops of lavender oil on your night-time pillow. Sweet dreams!

6. Communicate both your thoughts and your feelings clearly with your co-workers, friends, and loved ones. Remember that we all desire the same things—respect, kindness, appreciation, validation, and love. Keep the golden rule your default position in life, and treat others the way you like to be treated. Silently bless everyone in your life each day.

7. Lift your attitude *up* and see the best in everyone and everything. If you are facing a challenge, handle it with aplomb and élan and, at the same time, find opportunities to laugh and smile often. Both of these healthful activities firm your facial muscles and reduce stress. Laughter is life's elixir and our soul's smile. Cultivate a joyful attitude of gratitude. Attitude is the mind's paintbrush; it can color anything.

8. Choose to be responsible and accountable. Keep your word with yourself and others. Move past your excuses. Be disciplined. Discipline is the ability to carry out a resolution long after the mood or motivation has left you. Use the power that is yours to create what you desire and deserve—a fit and healthy body and a fulfilling, joyful, and peaceful life.

9. Love yourself and live peacefully. What better evidence of spiritual strength can we have than a peaceful mind and a loving heart? Champion your self-esteem, needs, and healthy self-boundaries. Create an empowered presence and invite joy, love, and peace into your life. Dream abundantly! Say *yes* to living your highest vision. Know that you deserve the very best of life's richest blessings. Celebrate yourself and life!

* * *

COMMITMENT TO HEALTH

Take a moment now and list all of the new healthful choices and salutary habits that you are going to make part of your new, transformed life. For example, in the space provided below, you might list things such as making fresh juices, getting more sleep, drinking more water, eating more raw foods, and making it a priority to focus on the positive.

_____   _____
_____   _____
_____   _____
_____   _____
_____   _____
_____   _____

This is also a good time to put into writing a list of all the new foods and kitchen tools that you are going to incorporate into your life. Use the space provided below.

_____   _____
_____   _____
_____   _____
_____   _____
_____   _____
_____   _____
_____   _____
_____   _____

Gratitude

As I strive to live my dream with as much heart and grace as possible, there are many people who have enriched my life and assisted me along my path. So I would like to take this opportunity to express my gratitude.

To Diane and David Beck, Susan Taylor Lennon, and James Michael Lennon for your expertise and support in helping me bring my vision to fruition.

To my family—June and Reid, Bryce and Tyler, June and Jamie, Tony and Ad, Suzi, and Jackie for blessing my life with so much loving kindness.

To Louise Hay, Jill Kramer, Reid Tracy, Beth Ellen Gustafson, Charles McStravick, Bridget Weeks, Carina Sammartino, Nancy Levin, Diane De Pasquale, Donna Abate, Jacqui Clark, Jessica Kelley, Stacey Smith, Margarete Nielsen, Richelle Zizian, Summer McStravick, Christy Salinas, Tricia Breidenthal, and the rest of the team at Hay House for giving life and energy to this book; and for helping to send its message of healthful, balanced living to as many people as possible worldwide.

To Lisa Ray, Lynn Carroll, Helen Guppy, Nick Colasanti, Violet Golden, Michael Provan, Dave and Alice Neighbors, Junia and John Chambers, Nick Lawrence, Rhio, Betty Wetzel, Bob Deskins, Donica Beath, Dianne Warren, Olin Idol, Diana Feinberg, Susan and Bill Kulick, Bonnie Ross, Kathleen Bureski, Gary Peattie, René Schmidt, Jamie Shourt, Elora Alden, Angela Colasanti, Eileen L. Hayden, Ralph Rudser, Rev. John Strickland, Denise Cook, Lynn Grudnik, Mamiko Matsuda, Jackie Day, Karen McGuire, Rev. Charles Taylor, Dr. Ronald Moy, Paulette Suzanne, Melissa Benzel, Dr. Helen Fincher, Jeanette Sinclair, Mary A. Tomlinson, Lori Bain, Rowena Gates, Victoria Moran, Lane Gray, and Steve Tyrell, people who add wonderful music, joy, and richness to my life.

ABOUT THE AUTHOR

For a woman with three of America's most ordinary names, **Susan Smith Jones, MS, PhD,** has certainly made extraordinary contributions in the fields of optimum health, fitness, longevity, and human potential. Selected as one of ten "Healthy American Fitness Leaders"[1] by the President's Council on Physical Fitness & Sports, Susan is an award-winning writer and advice columnist. She has authored hundreds of magazine articles, numerous audio programs, and 17 books, including *Choose to Live Peacefully, Wired to Meditate, Choose to Live Fully, Be Healthy—Stay Balanced, Vegetable Soup/The Fruit Bowl* (co-authored with Dianne Warren—for children ages 1–9), and *Celebrate Life!*, as well as her upcoming books, *The Healing Power of NATUREFOODS—Volumes 2 and 3,* published by Hay House.

Susan appears regularly in the pages and on the covers of national and international publications, and is a frequent guest on radio and television talk shows around the country. For 30 years, she taught students, staff, and faculty at UCLA how to be healthy and fit. On her frequent lecture tours, she discusses how to look younger and live longer; boost immunity and energy; minimize stress and maximize joy; prevent and alleviate disease; use food as medicine; set up a healthful kitchen; create meals that rejuvenate the body; detoxify the body with

---

[1]Previous winners include Lance Armstrong, the late Ronald Reagan, former UCLA basketball coach John Wooden, Kathy Smith, Denise Austin, Richard Simmons, and Jack LaLanne.

157

whole foods and fresh juices; make tasty blender meals in seconds; raise healthy children; and bring a sacred balance into your body and life.

An acclaimed holistic health and lifestyle coach, private culinary instructor, and whole-foods chef, Susan works with discerning clients around the world. She creates menus and rejuvenation programs designed to support and complement the needs of her individual clients, as well as the participants at her specialized holistic health retreats. In addition, she serves as a recipe developer and new-product consultant for the health industry.

Susan's inspiring message and innovative techniques for achieving total health in body, mind, and spirit have won her a grateful and enthusiastic following and have put her in constant demand internationally as a health and fitness consultant and motivational speaker (lectures, workshops, and keynote presentations) for community, corporate, and religious/spiritual groups. She also is founder and president of Health Unlimited, a Los Angeles–based consulting firm dedicated to the advancement of peaceful, balanced living and health education. (See her website below for more information about scheduling workshops and appearances.)

Many years ago, when a devastating car accident fractured Susan's back so severely that doctors told her she would never again be physically active and would live a life of chronic pain, she proved her doctors wrong. Her miraculous recovery proved to her that we all have within ourselves everything we need to live our lives to the fullest. She now regularly participates in a variety of fitness activities, including hiking, weight training, in-line skating, biking, Pilates, horseback riding, and yoga. A film enthusiast, Susan enjoys spending her free time going to movies, especially any starring Steve Martin, Helen Mirren, Denzel Washington, or Meryl Streep; she also appreciates films featuring the music of Steve Tyrell. A gifted teacher, Susan brings together modern research and ageless wisdom in all her work. She resides in West Los Angeles.

For more information, visit:

www.SusanSmithJones.com

* * *

"There is a principle which is a bar against information,
which is proof against all argument, and
which cannot fail to keep a man in everlasting ignorance.
That principle is Contempt prior to investigation."
—Herbert Spencer

* * *

"Every day brings a chance for you
to draw in a breath,
kick off your shoes,
and dance."
—Oprah Winfrey

* * *

We hope you enjoyed this Hay House book.
If you would like to receive a free catalogue featuring additional
Hay House books and products, or if you would like information
about the Hay Foundation, please contact:

Hay House UK Ltd
292B Kensal Rd • London W10 5BE
Tel: (44) 20 8962 1230; Fax: (44) 20 8962 1239
www.hayhouse.co.uk

❋❋❋

Published and distributed in the United States of America by:
Hay House, Inc. • PO Box 5100 • Carlsbad, CA 92018-5100
Tel.: (1) 760 431 7695 or (1) 800 654 5126;
Fax: (1) 760 431 6948 or (1) 800 650 5115
www.hayhouse.com

Published and distributed in Australia by:
Hay House Australia Ltd • 18/36 Ralph St • Alexandria NSW 2015
Tel.: (61) 2 9669 4299; Fax: (61) 2 9669 4144
www.hayhouse.com.au

Published and distributed in the Republic of South Africa by:
Hay House SA (Pty) Ltd • PO Box 990 • Witkoppen 2068
Tel./Fax: (27) 11 467 8904 • www.hayhouse.co.za

Published and distributed in India by:
Hay House Publishers India • Muskaan Complex • Plot No.3
B-2 • Vasant Kunj • New Delhi – 110 070.
Tel.: (91) 11 41761620; Fax: (91) 11 41761630.
www.hayhouse.co.in

Distributed in Canada by:
Raincoast • 9050 Shaughnessy St • Vancouver, BC V6P 6E5
Tel.: (1) 604 323 7100; Fax: (1) 604 323 2600

❋❋❋

Sign up via the Hay House UK website to receive the Hay House
online newsletter and stay informed about what's going on with
your favourite authors. You'll receive bimonthly announcements
about discounts and offers, special events, product highlights,
free excerpts, giveaways, and more!
www.hayhouse.co.uk